THE STORY OF CANCER
Volume 4

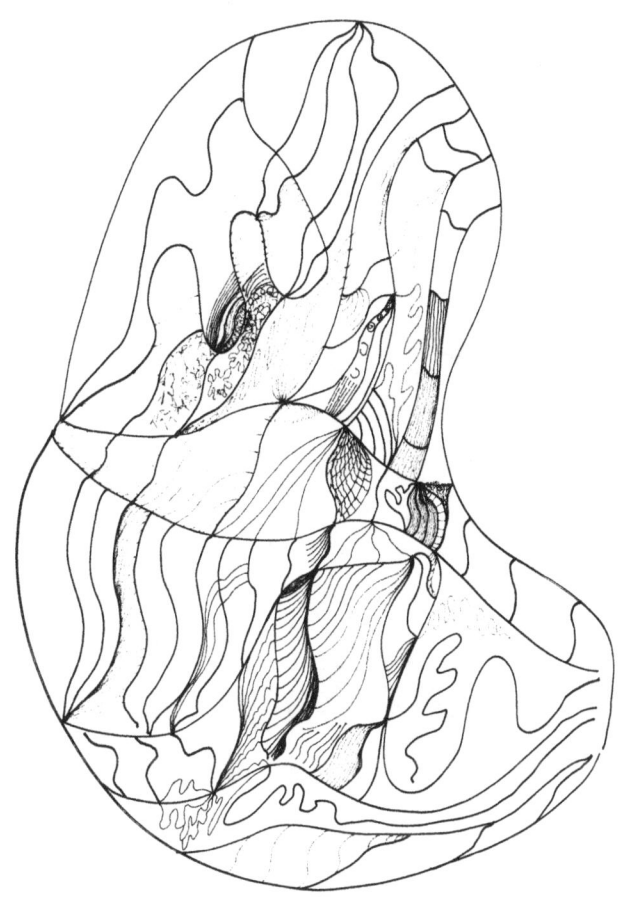

Camilia MacPherson, Ph.D., D.Th.
2016

INTRODUCTION

This is the Story of Cancer using Automatic Drawings and Surreal Art. It is part of a continuous document written in 7 volumes.

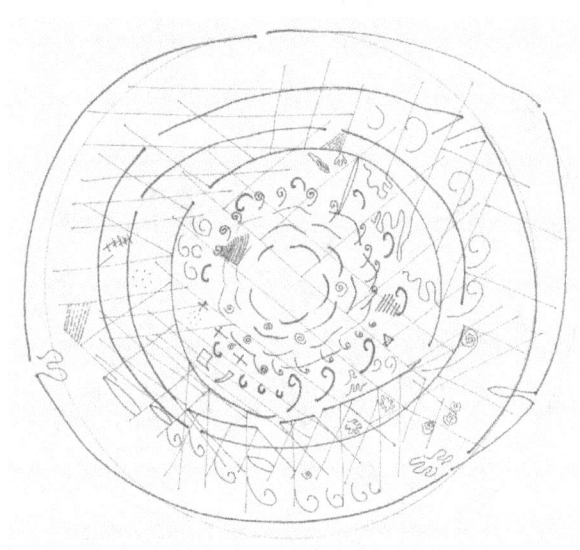

ISBN-13: 9781530545667
ISBN-10: 1530545668
Email: tamaracpublishers@icloud.com

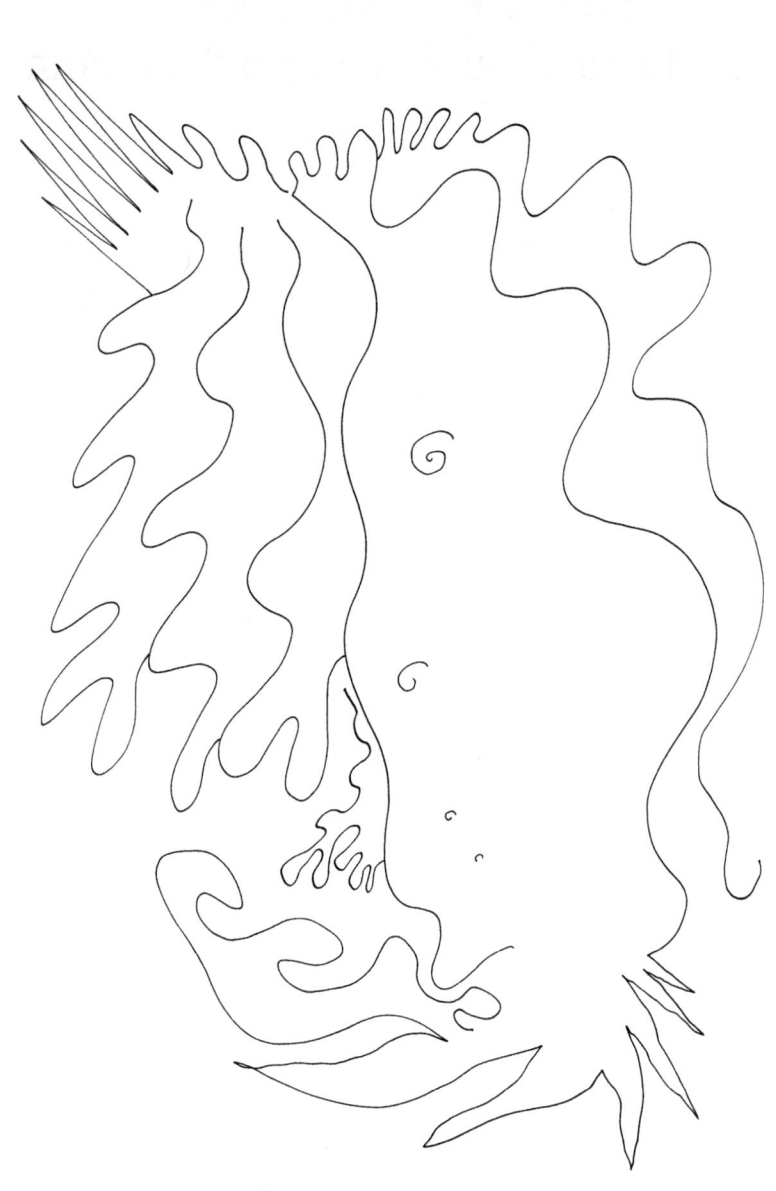

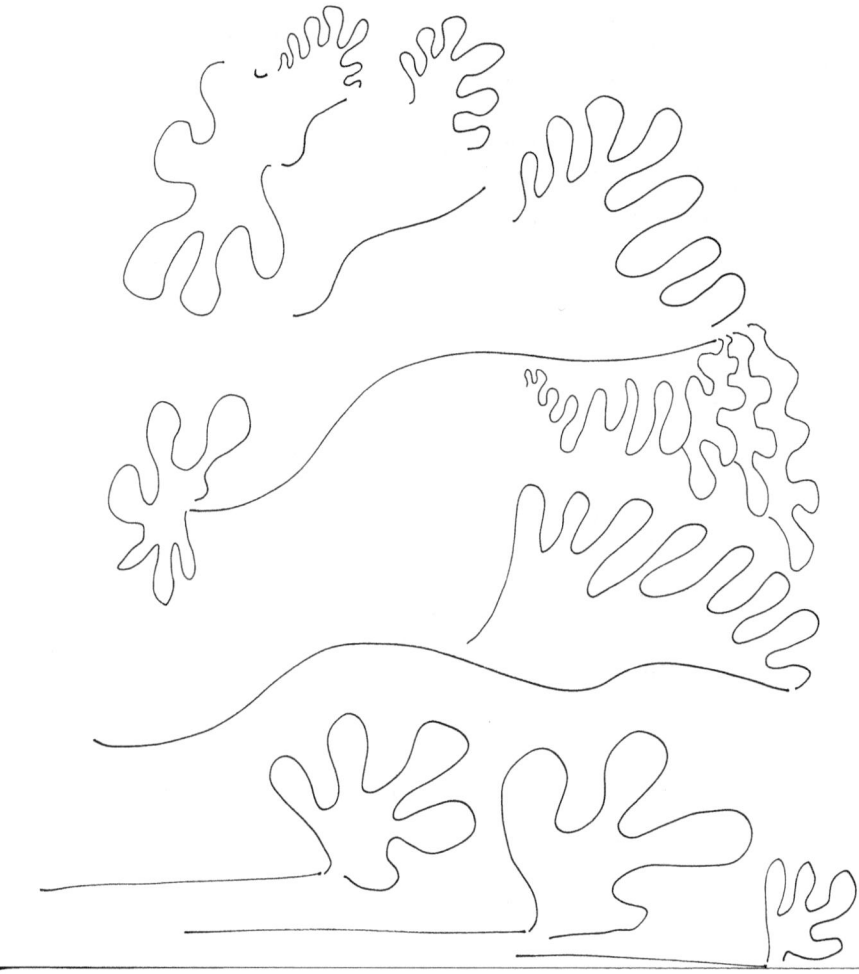

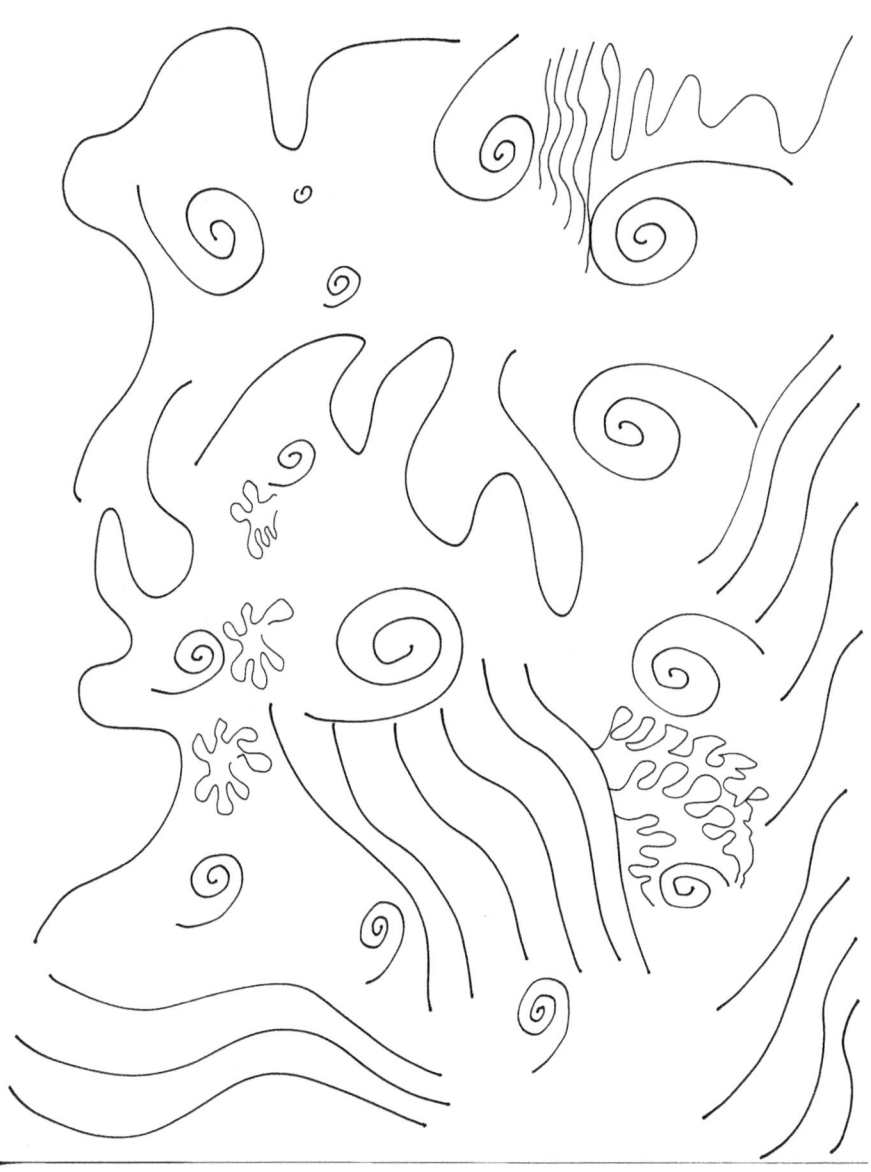

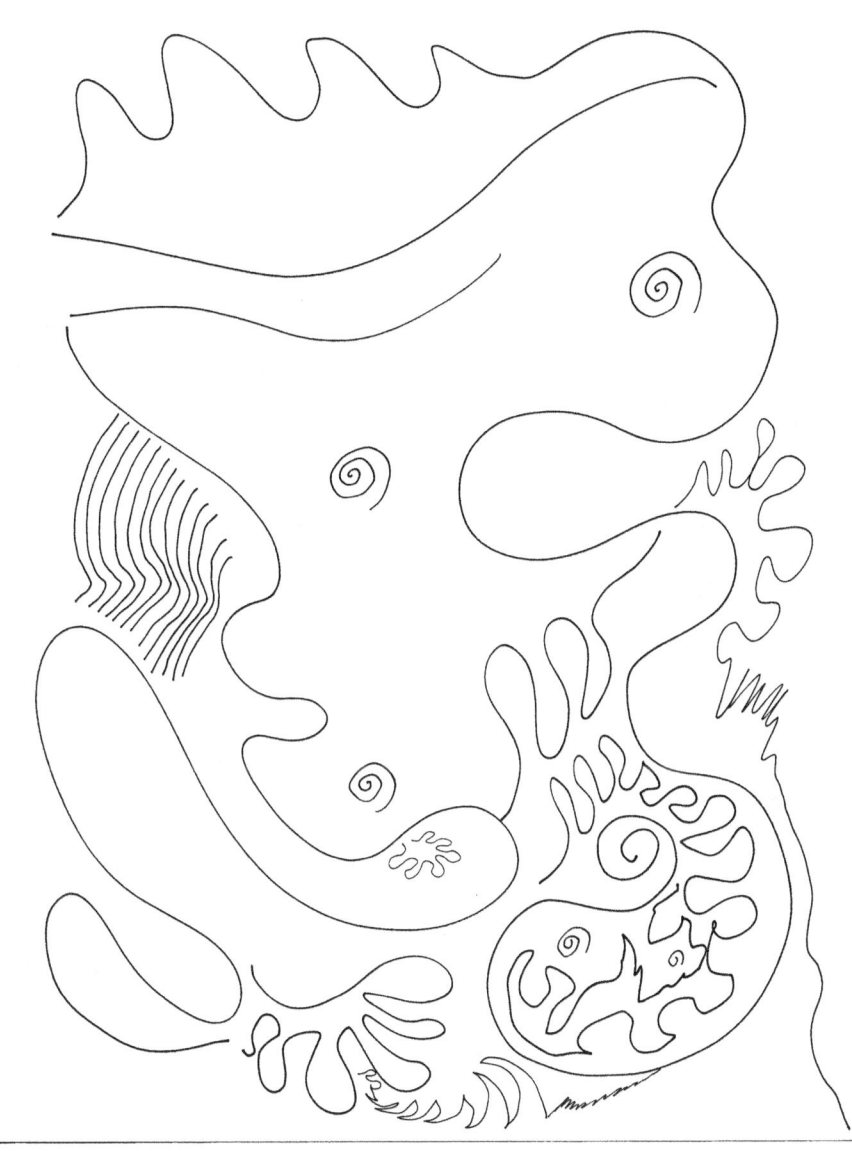

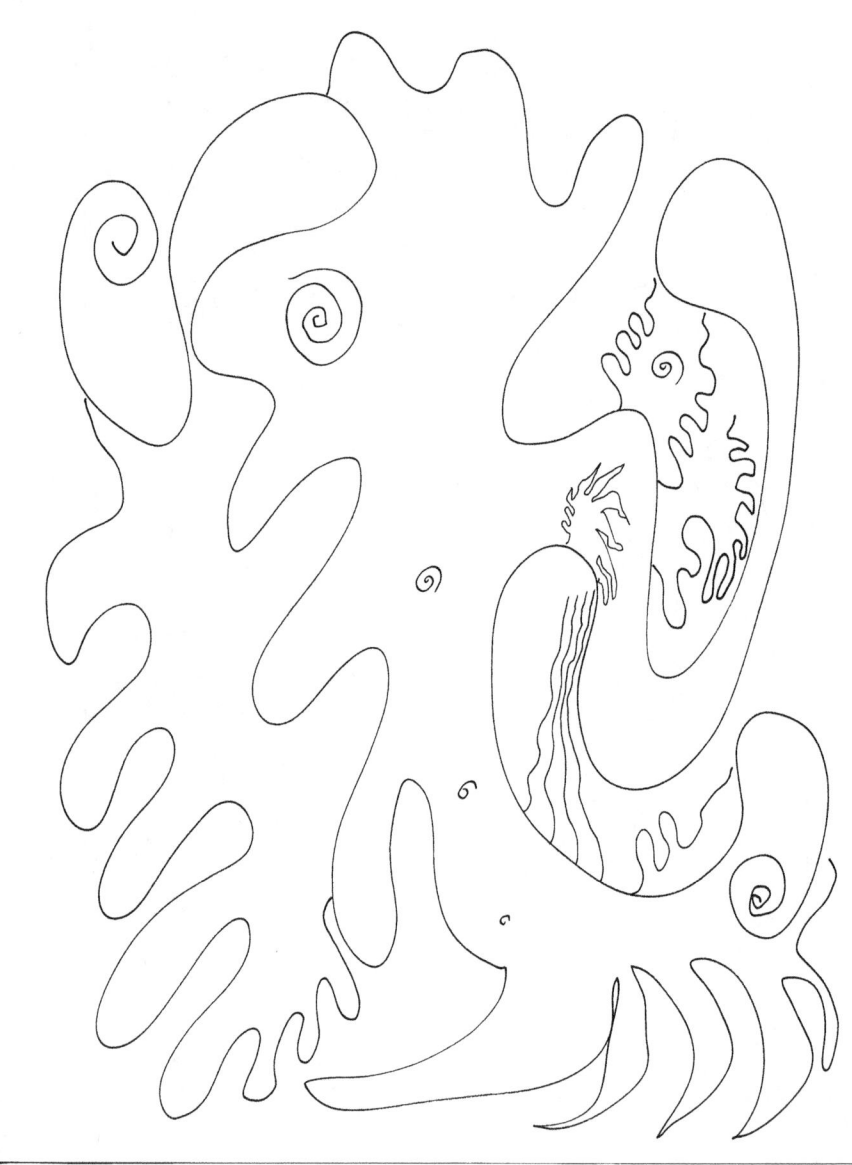

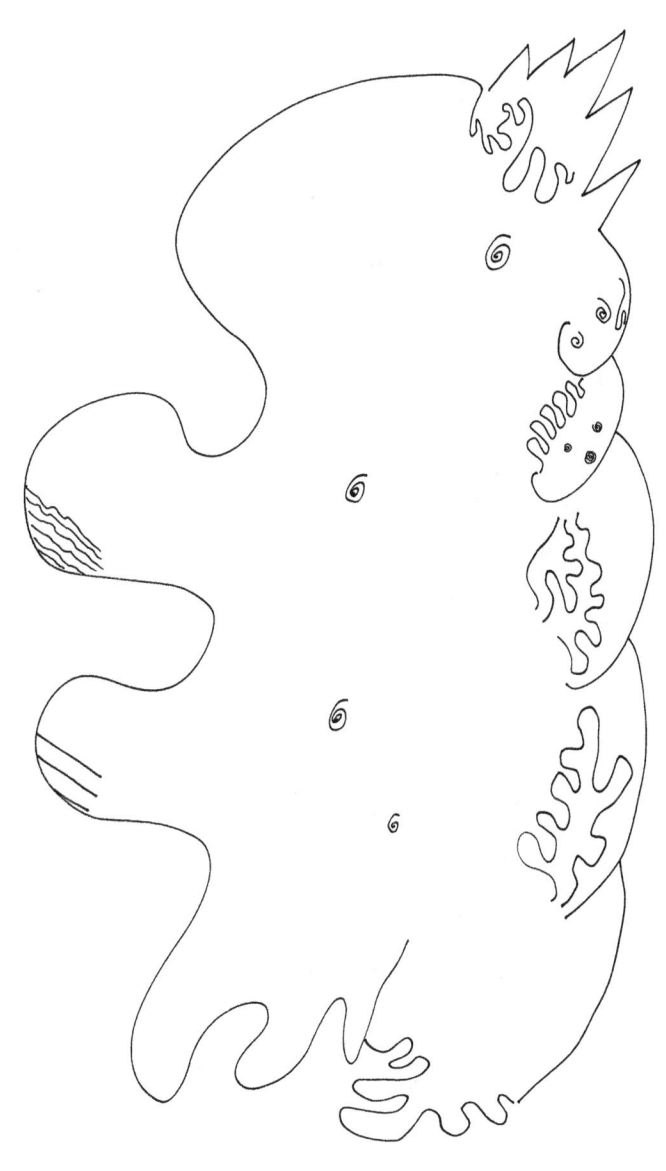

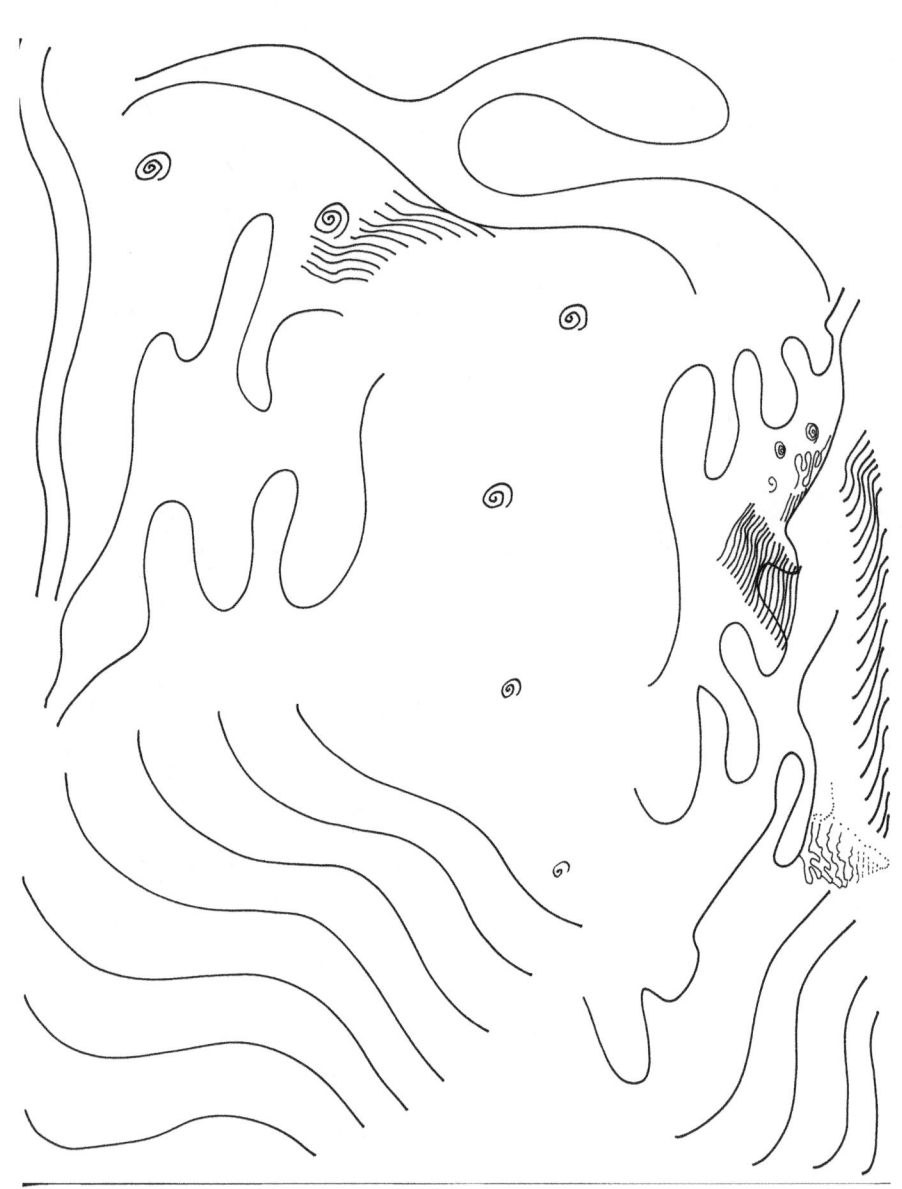

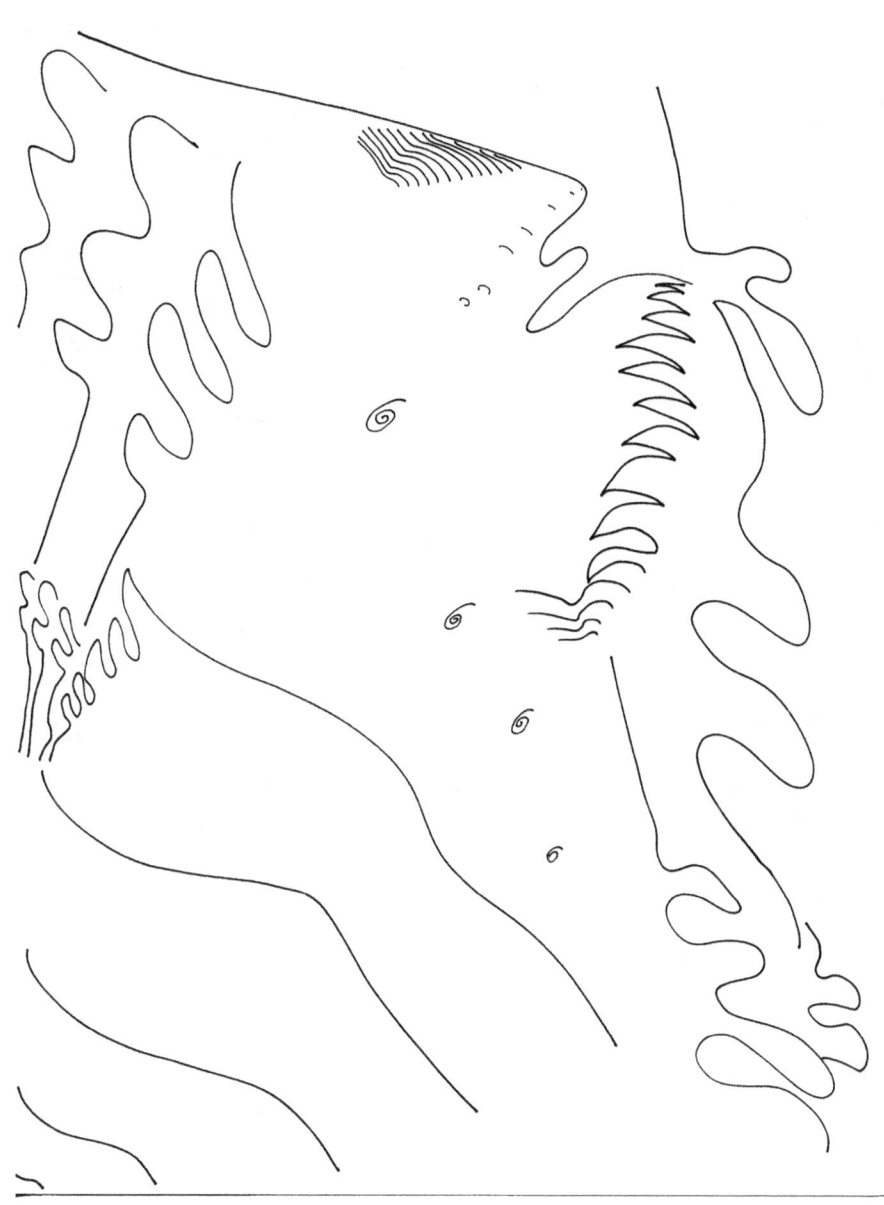

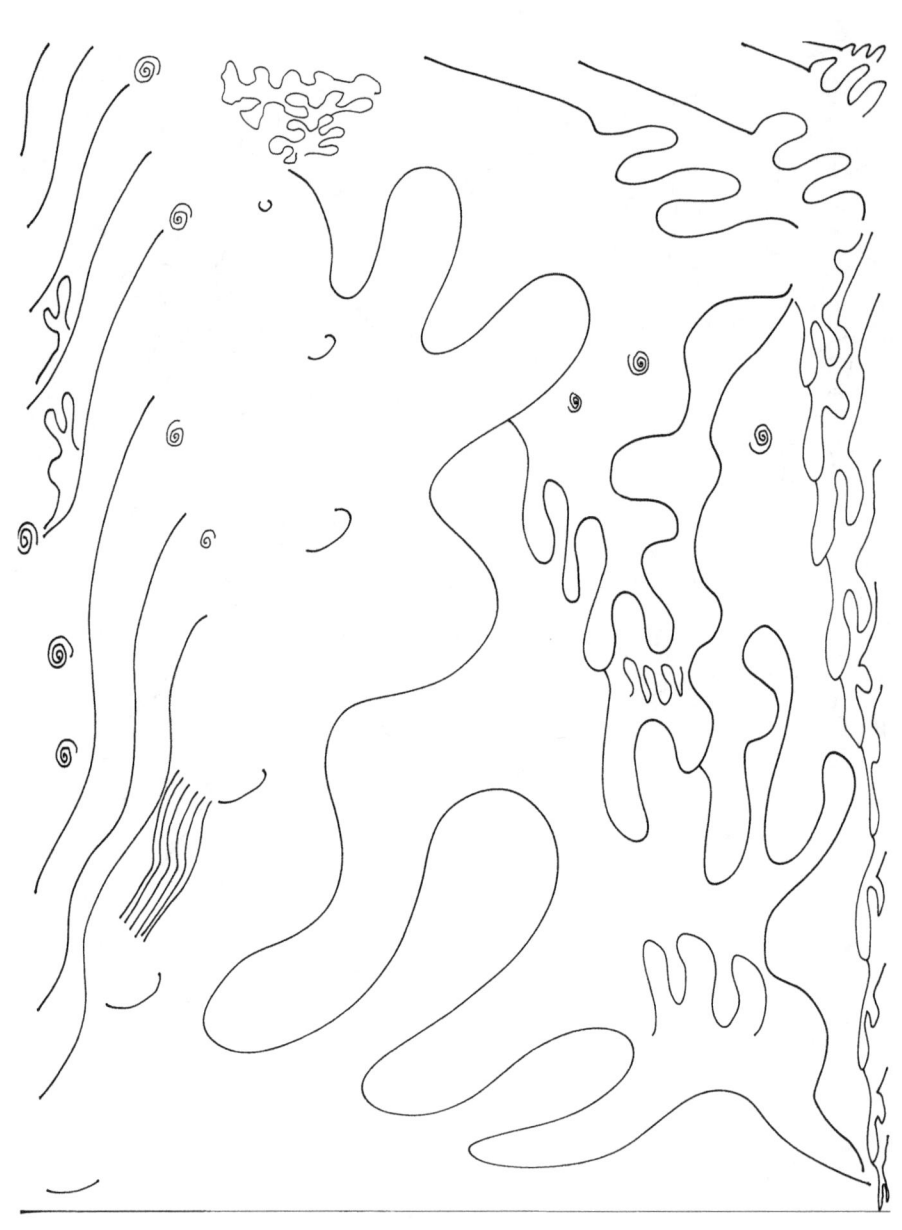

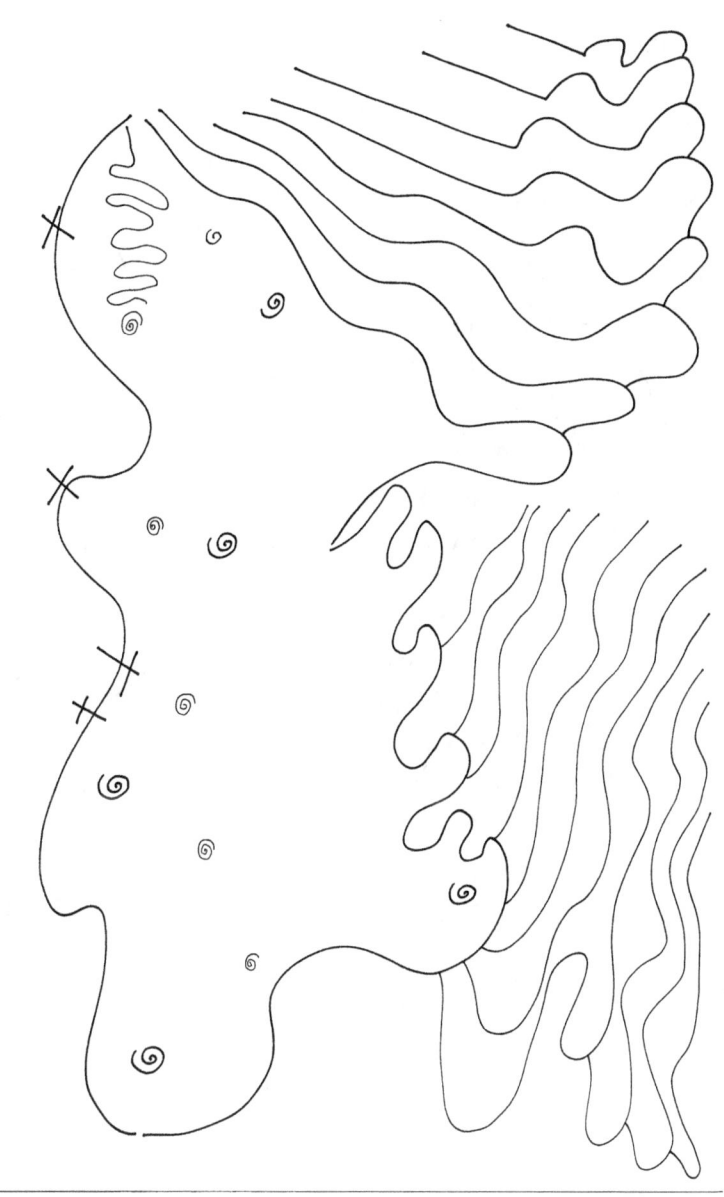

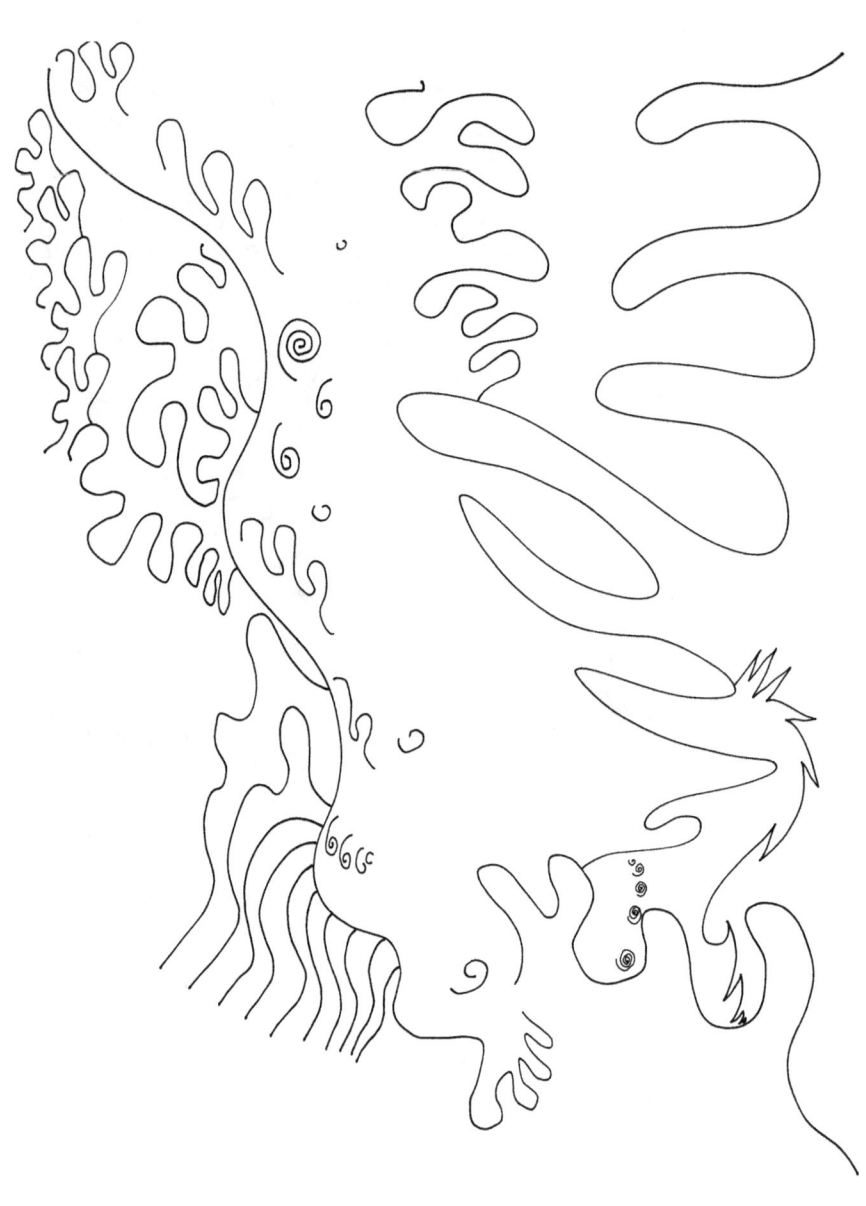

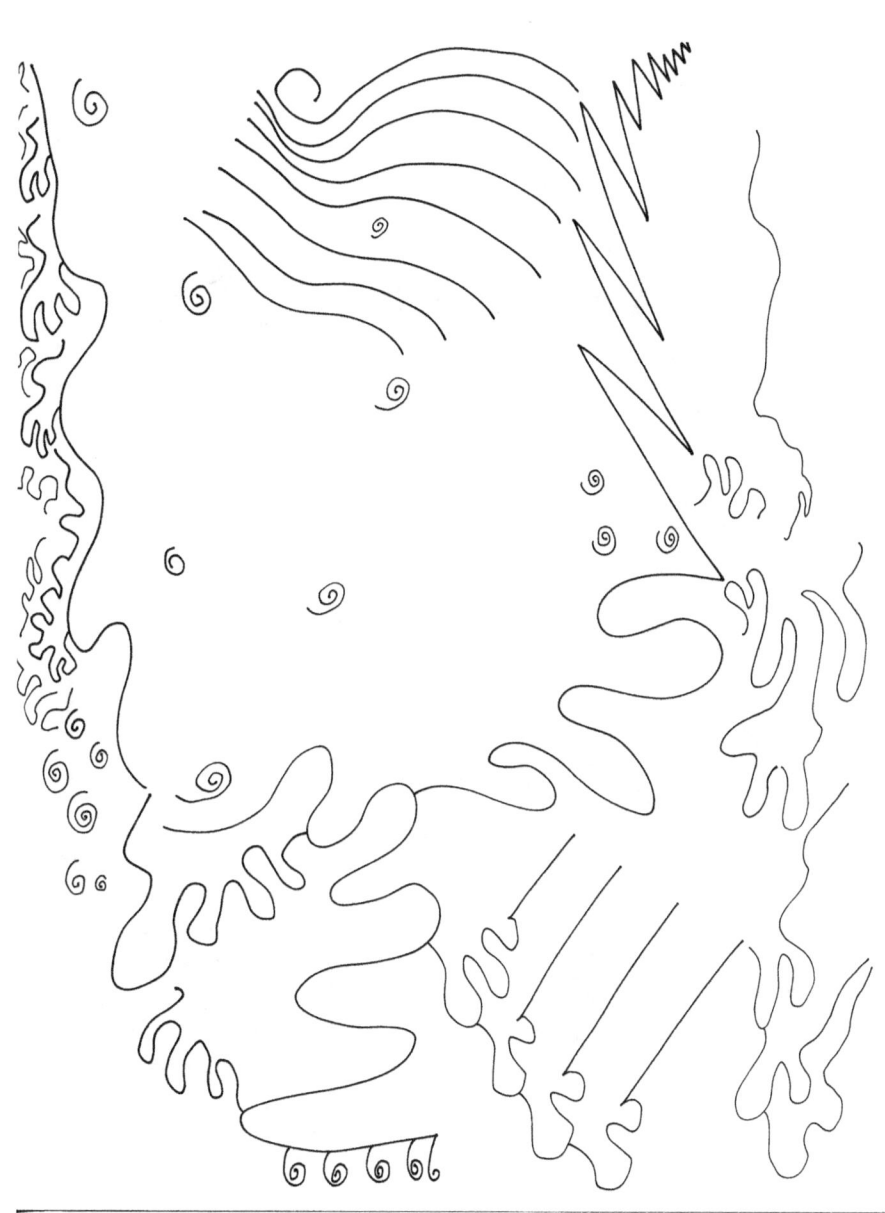

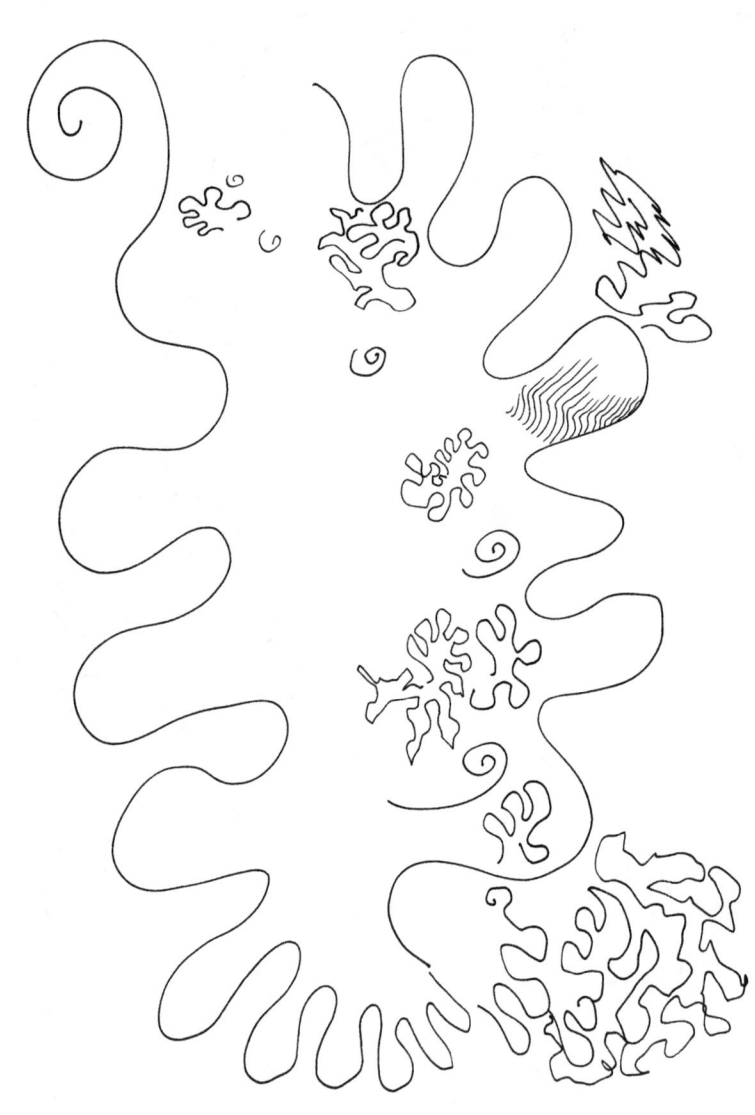

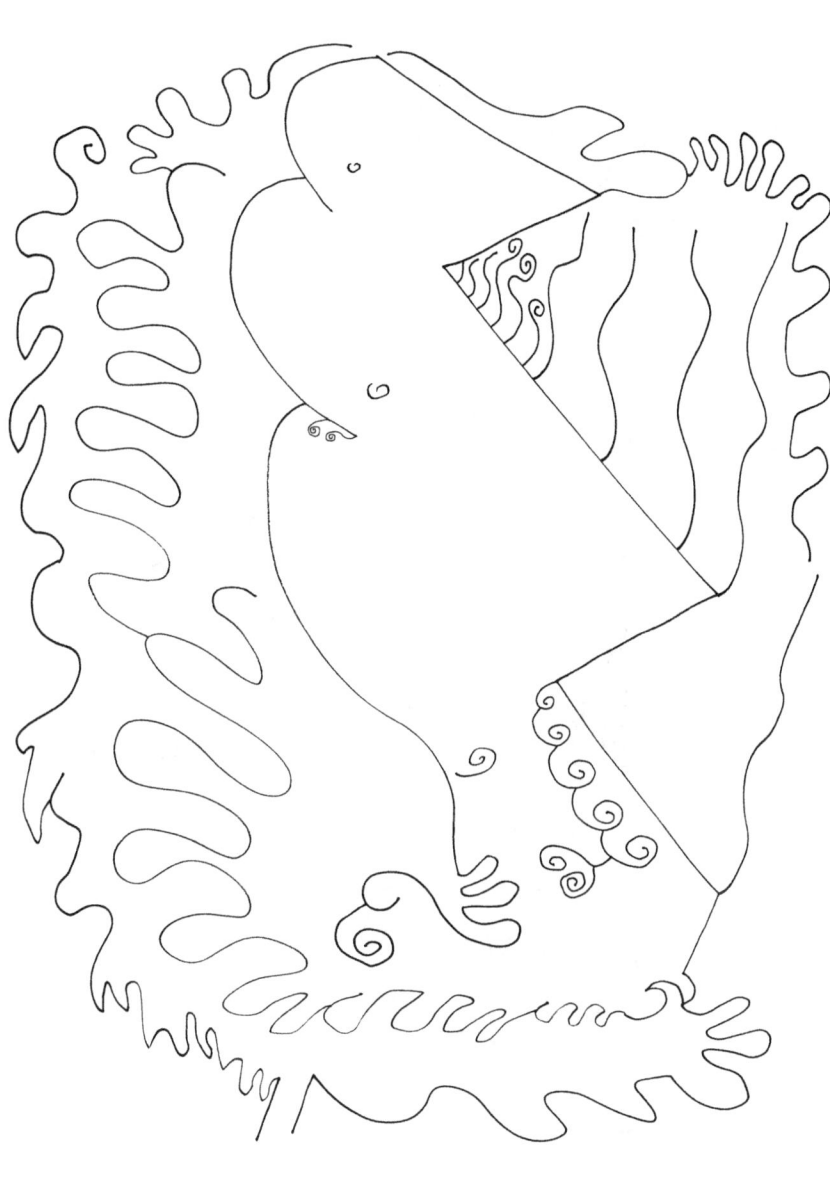

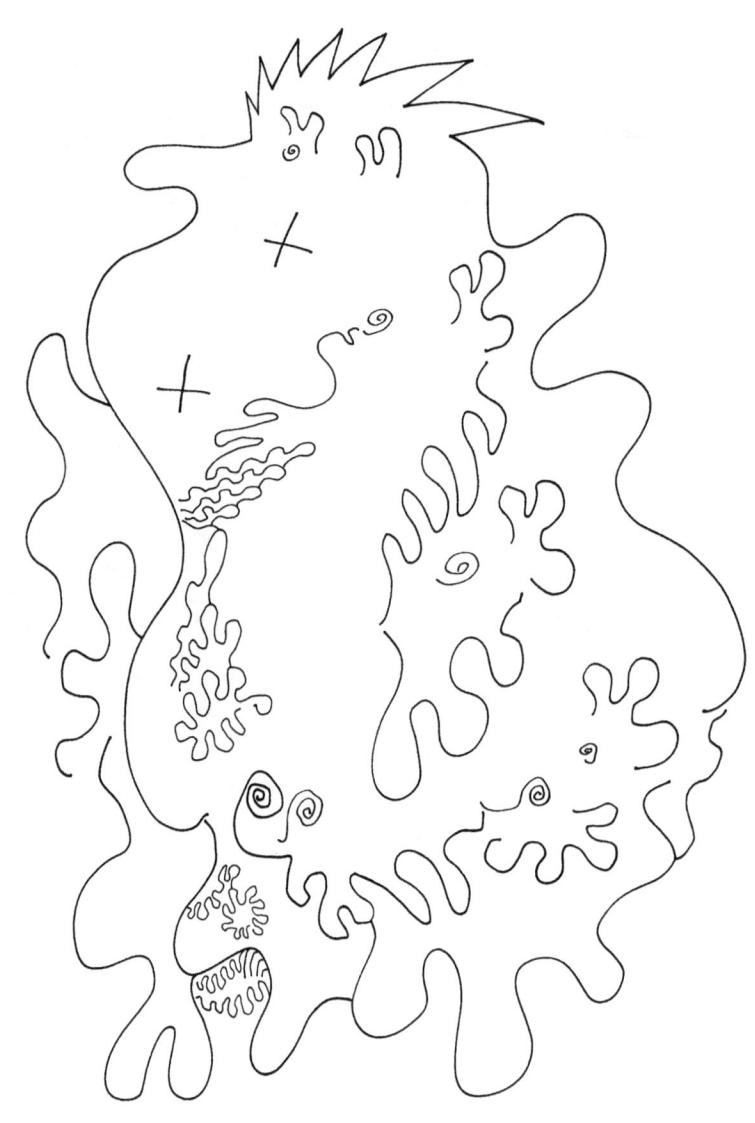

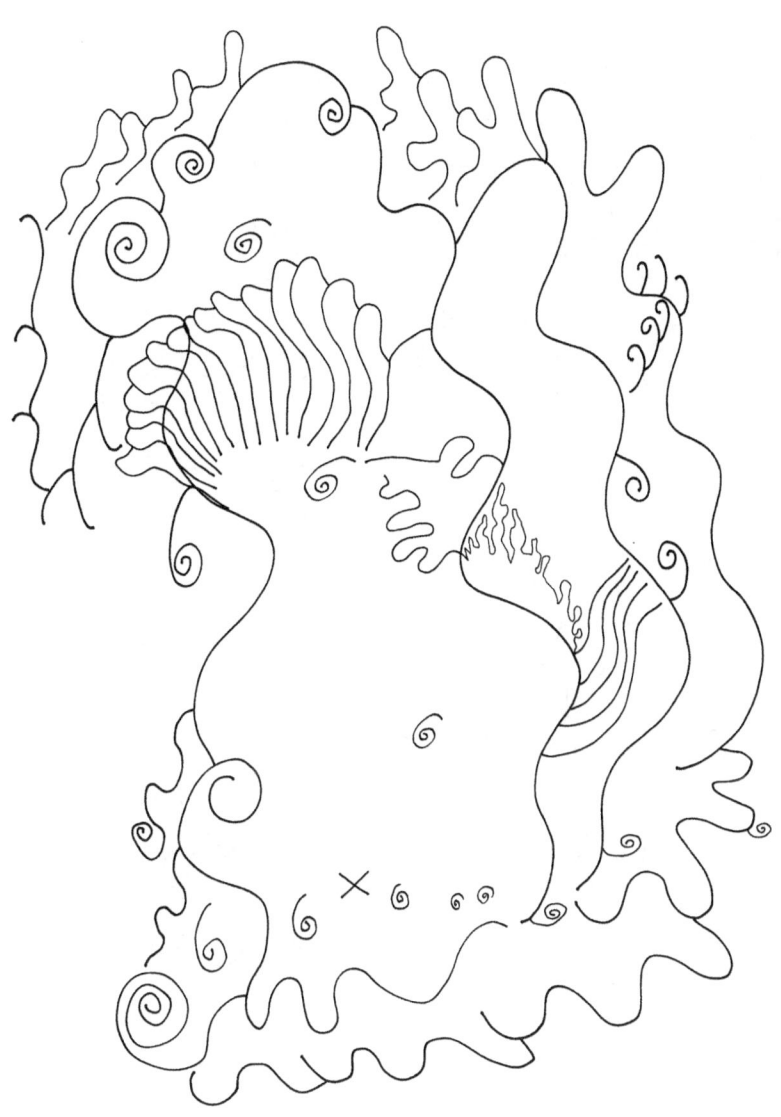

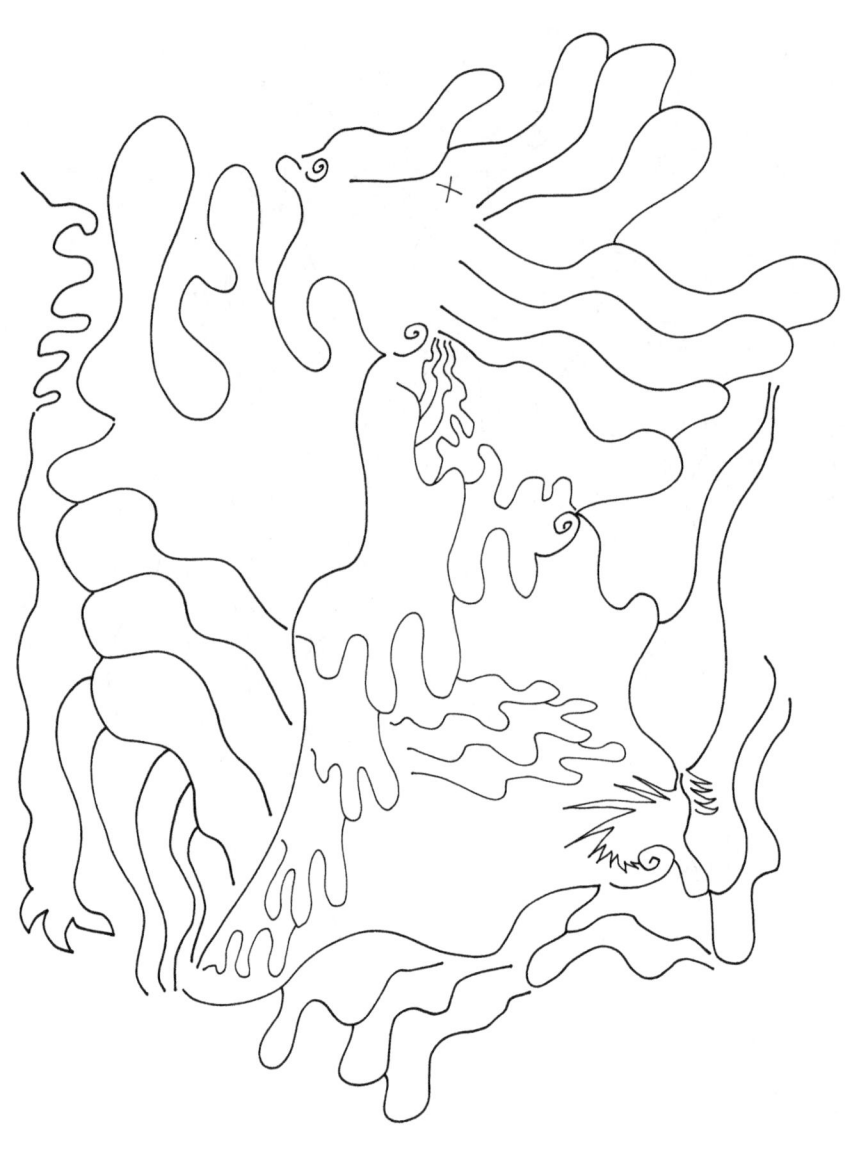

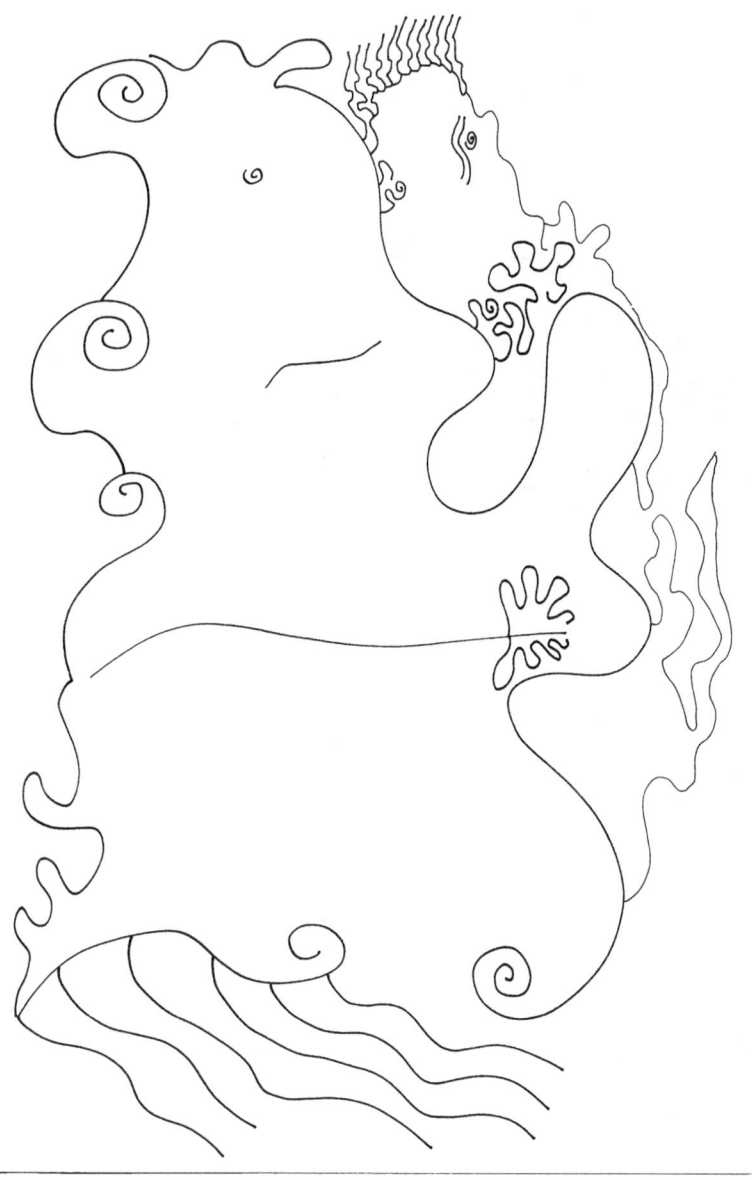

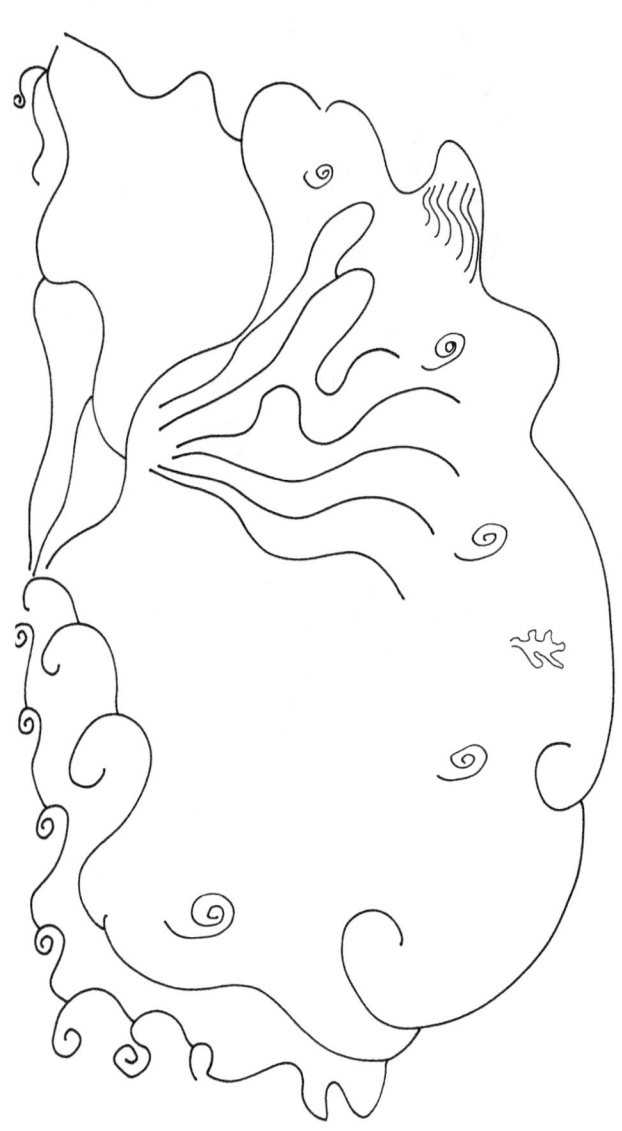

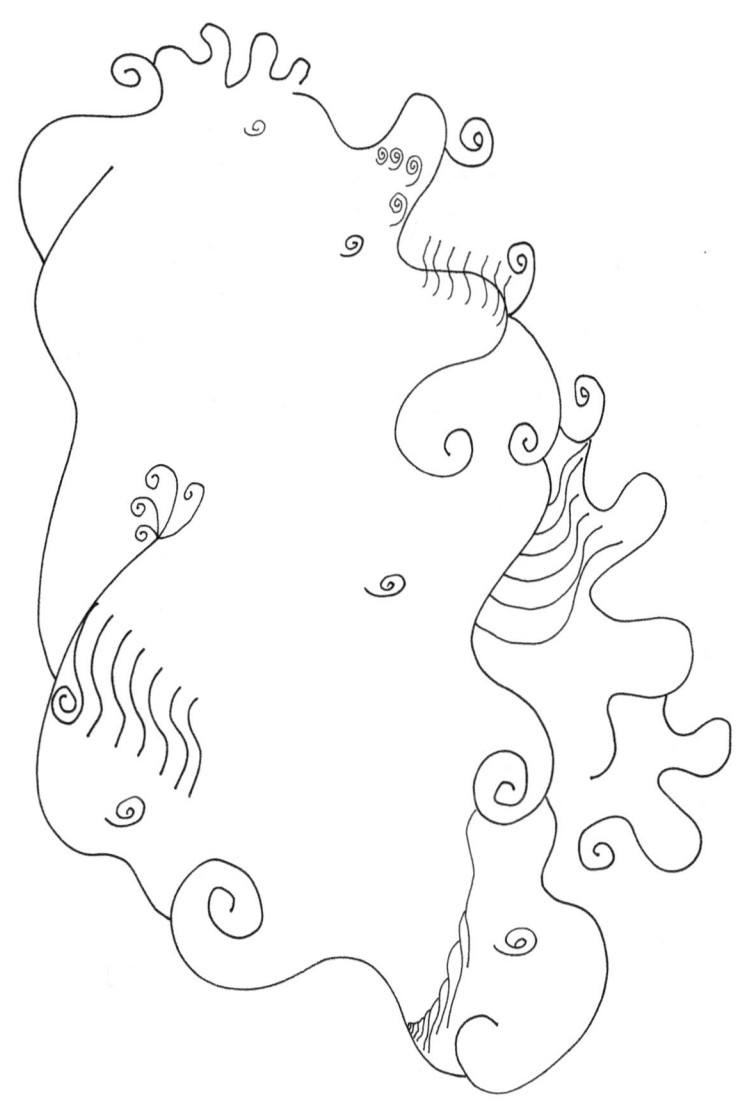

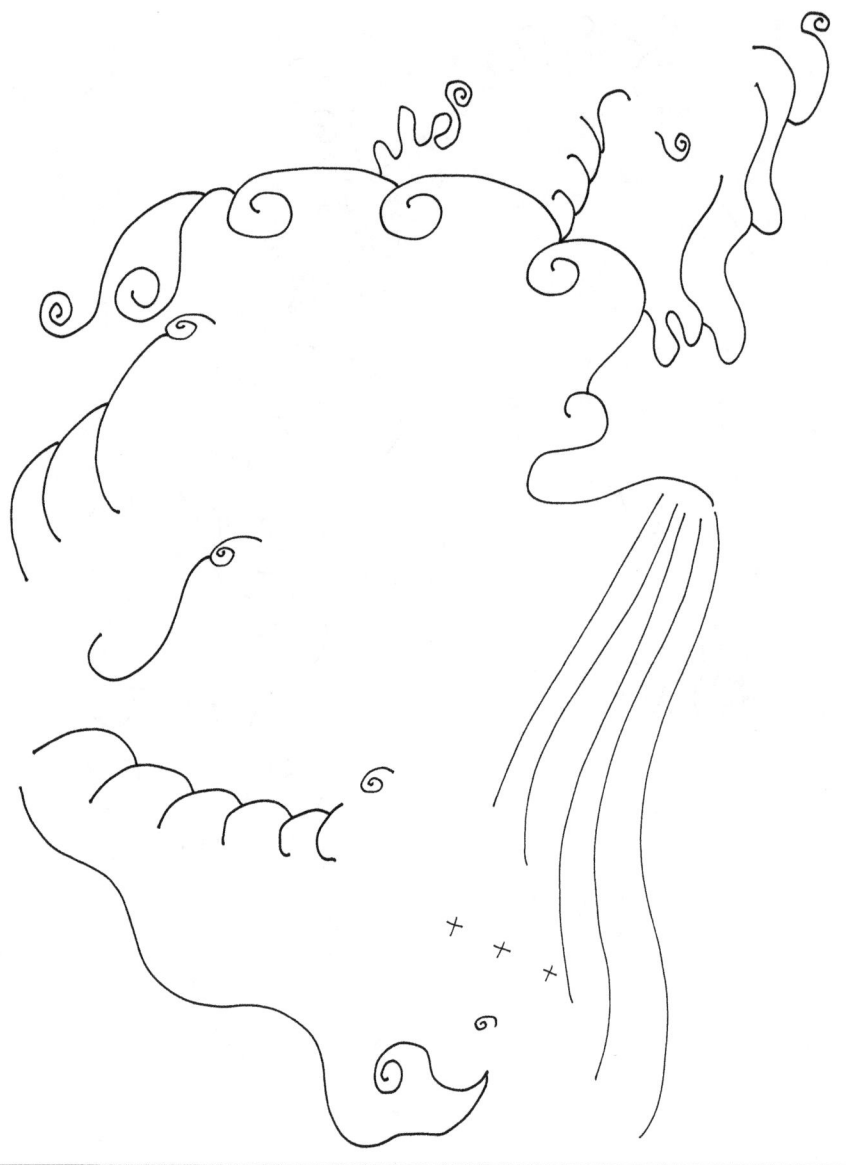

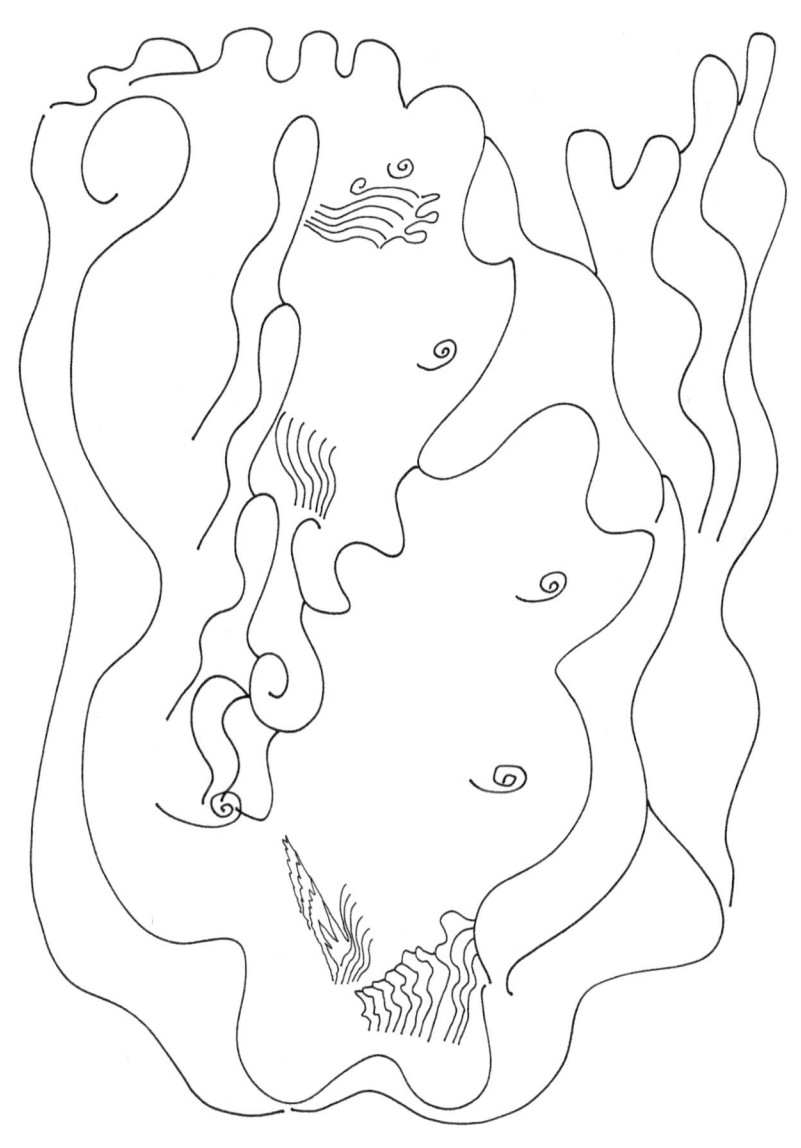

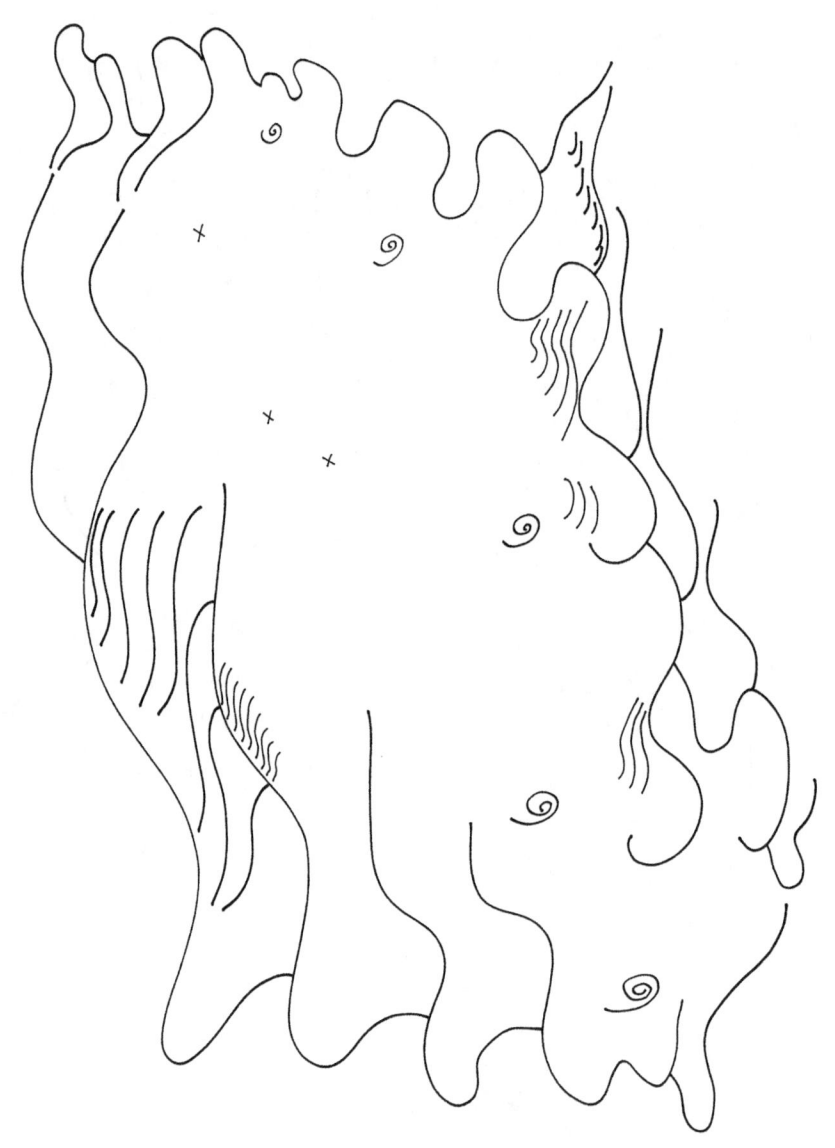

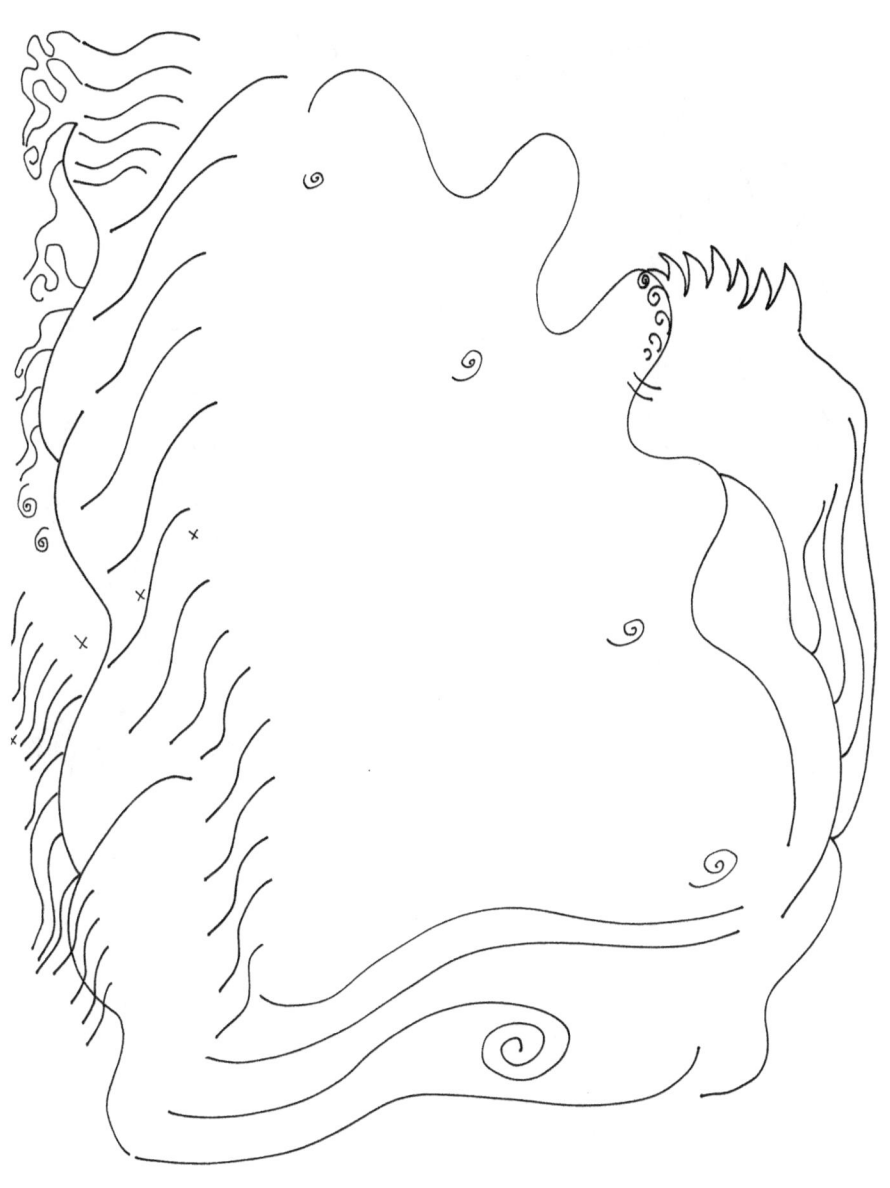

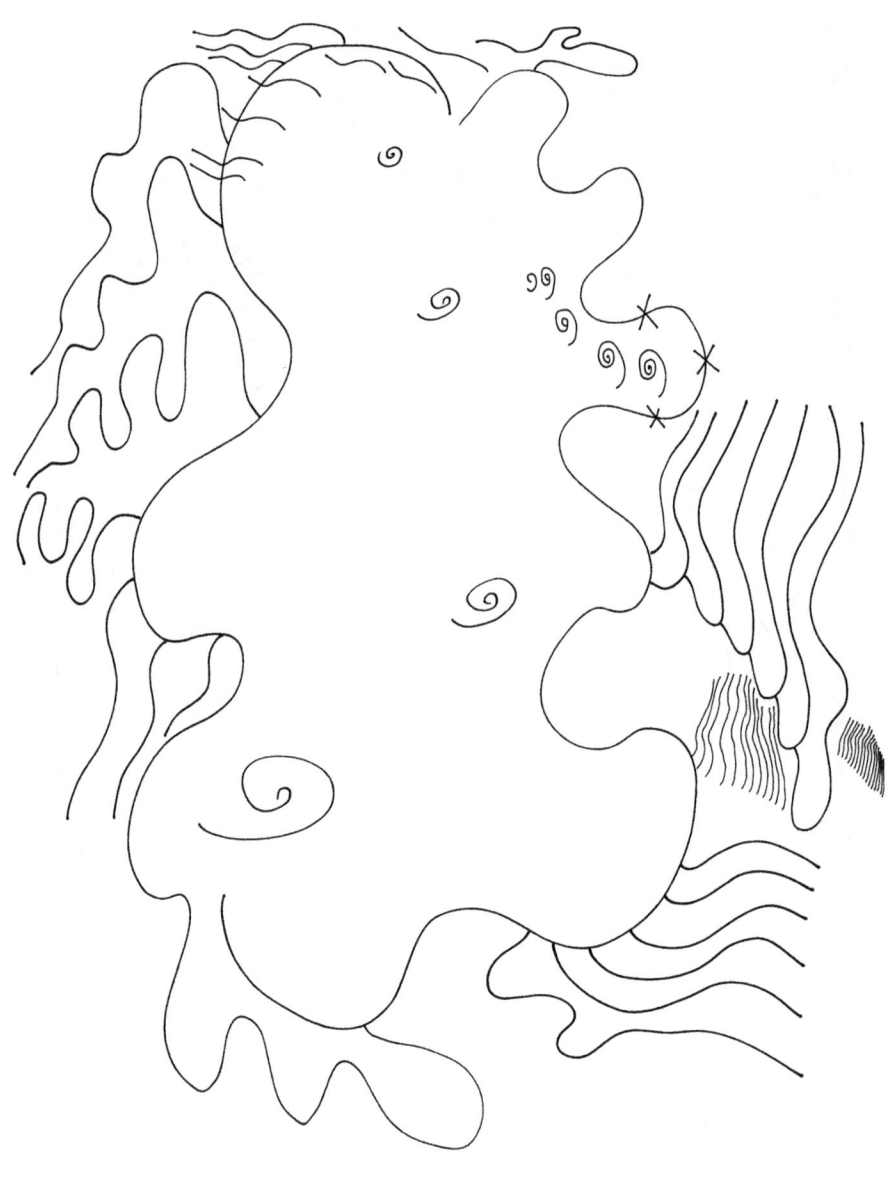

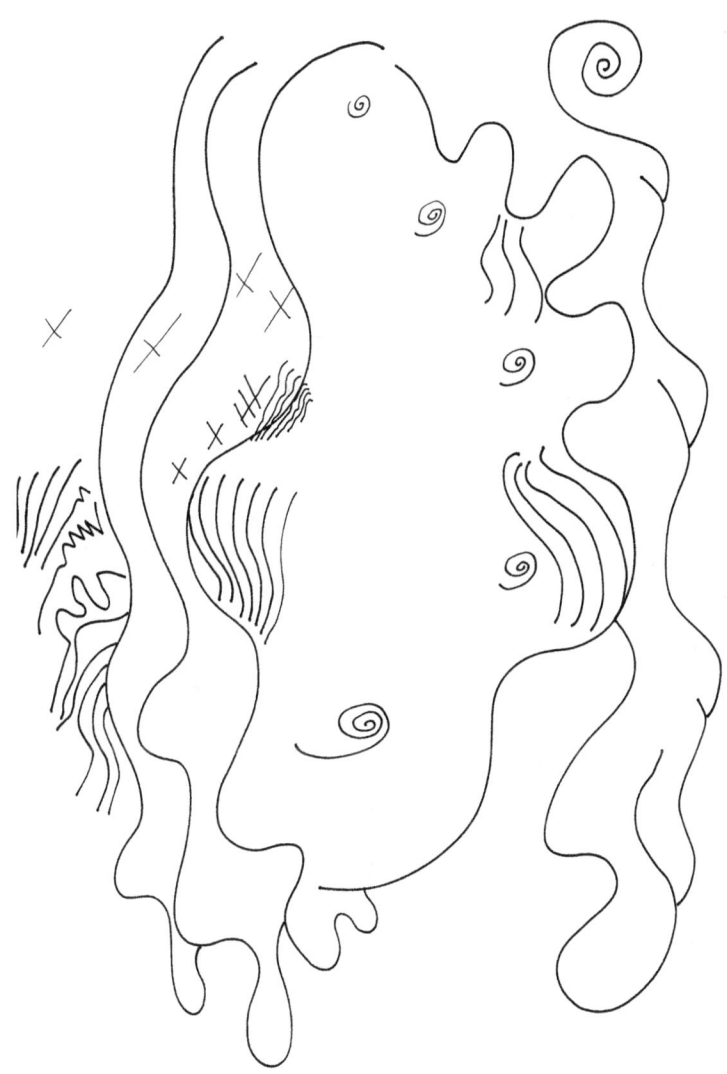

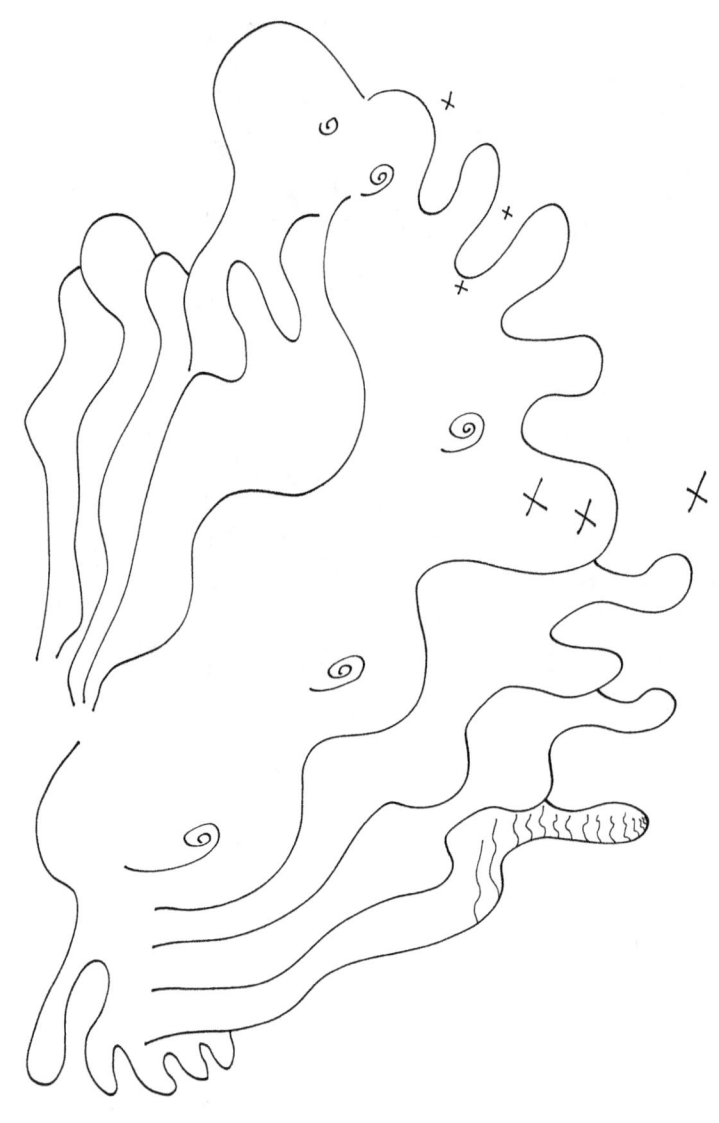

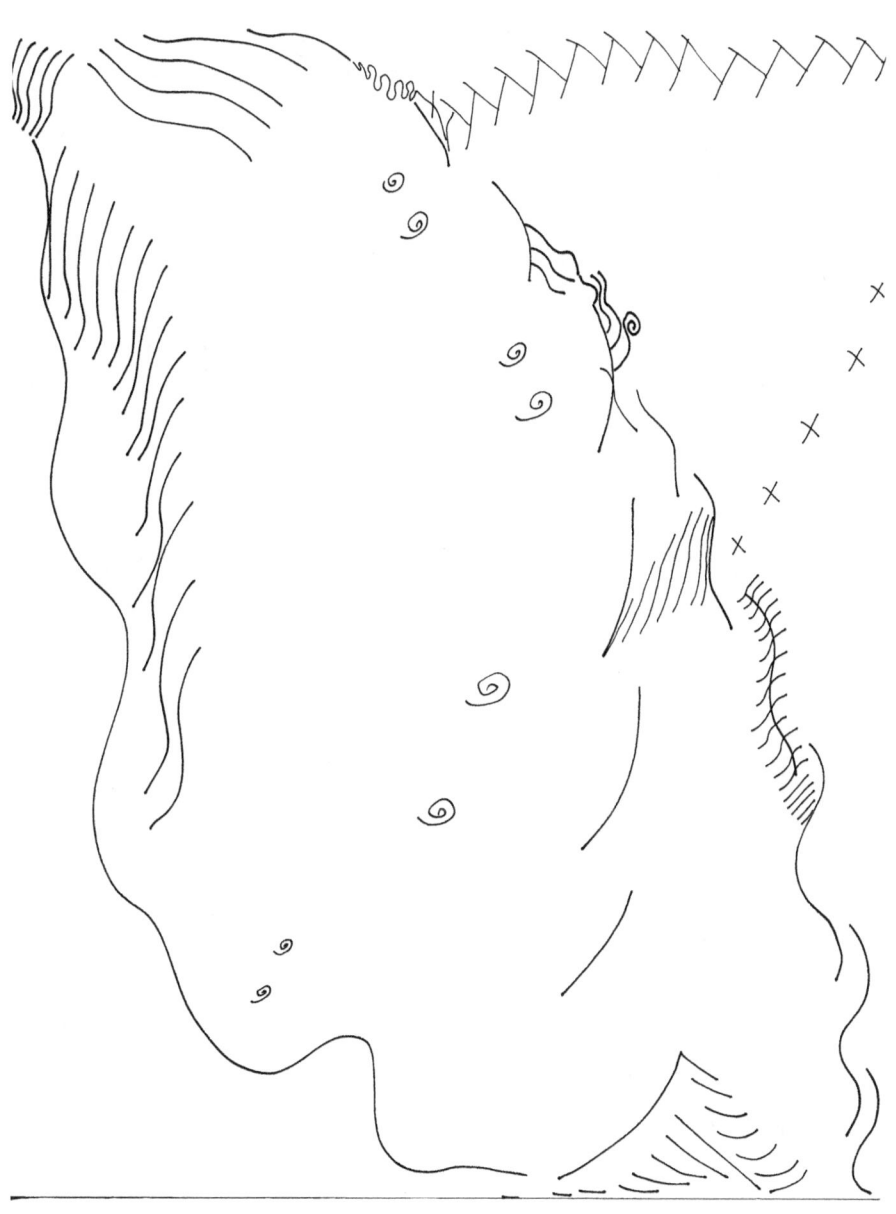

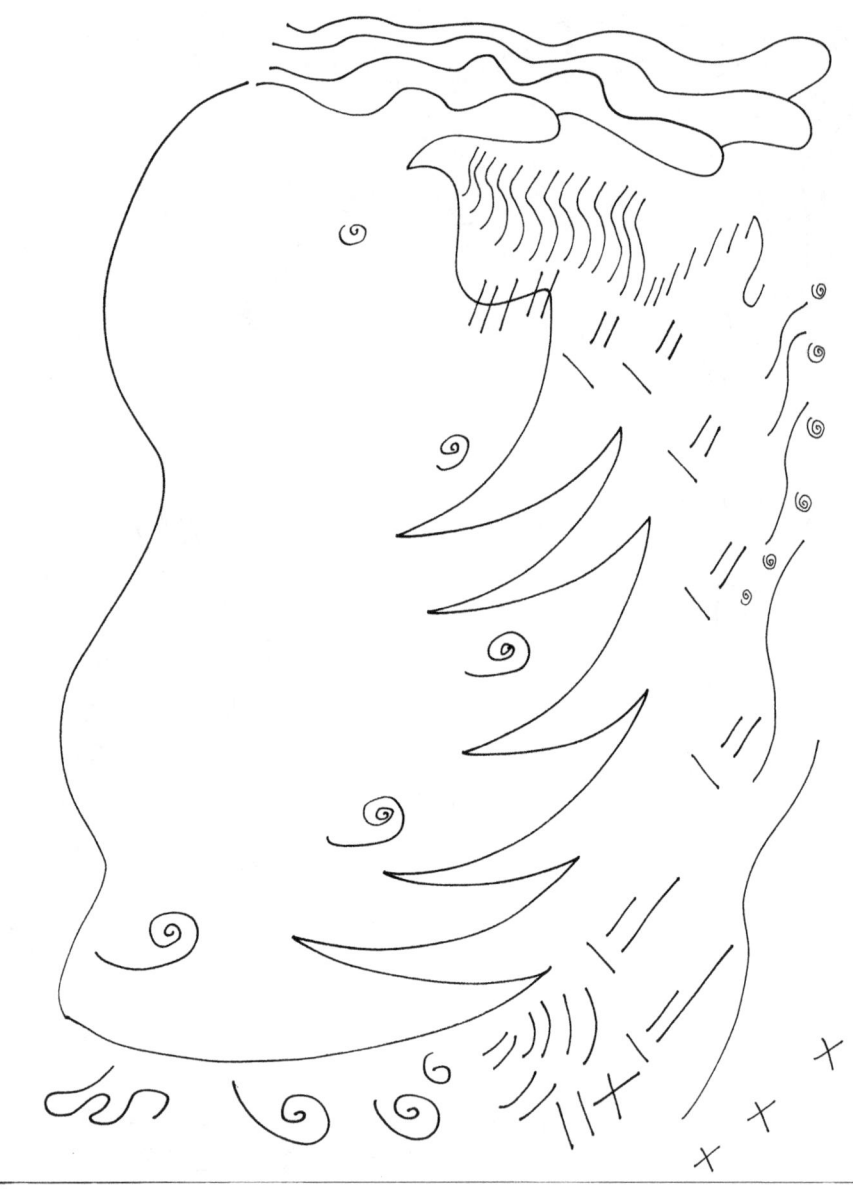

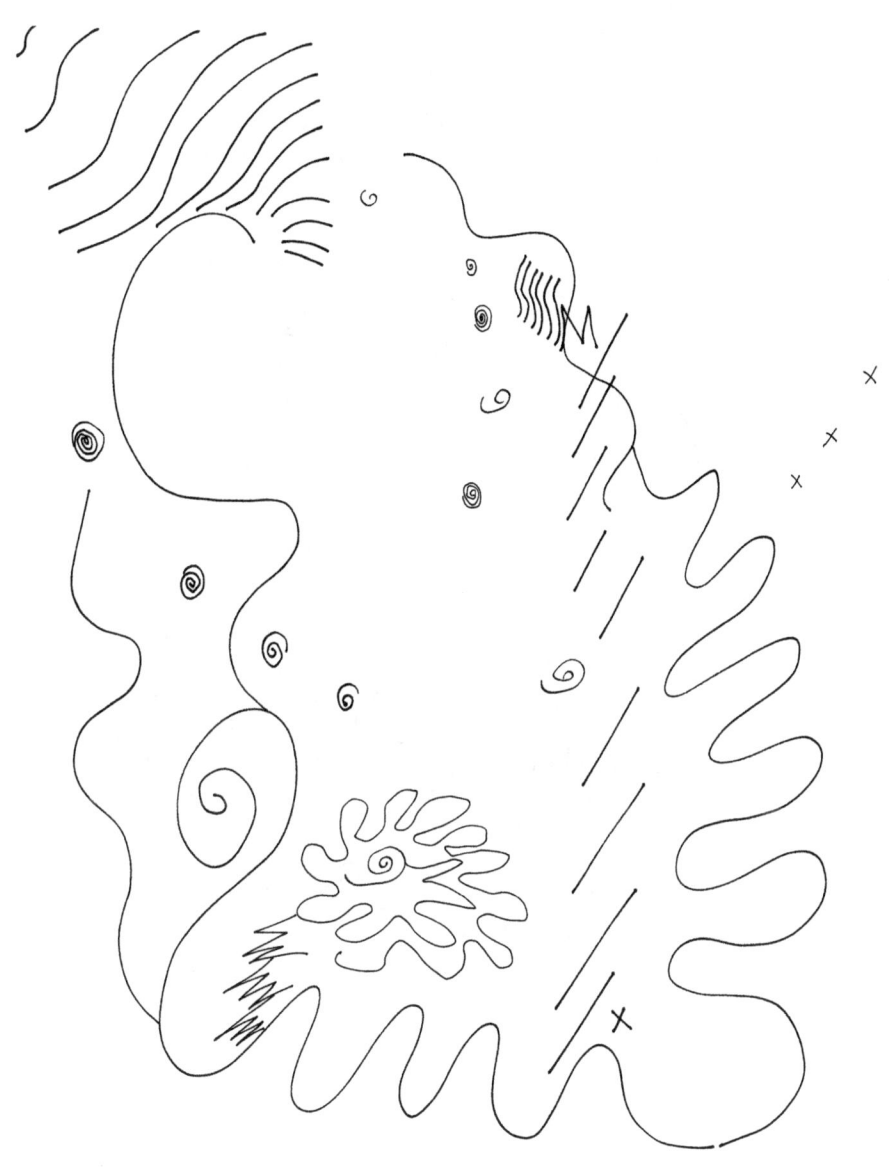

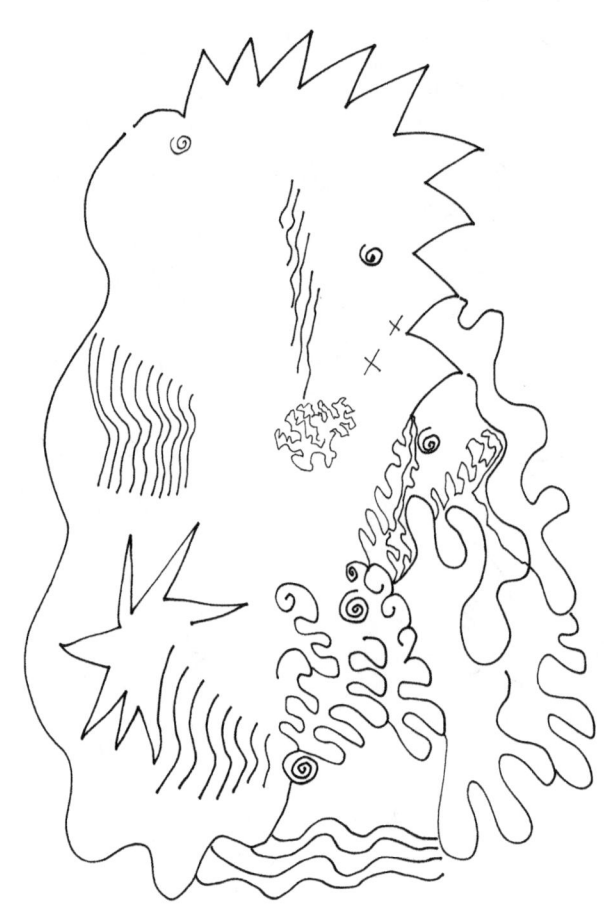

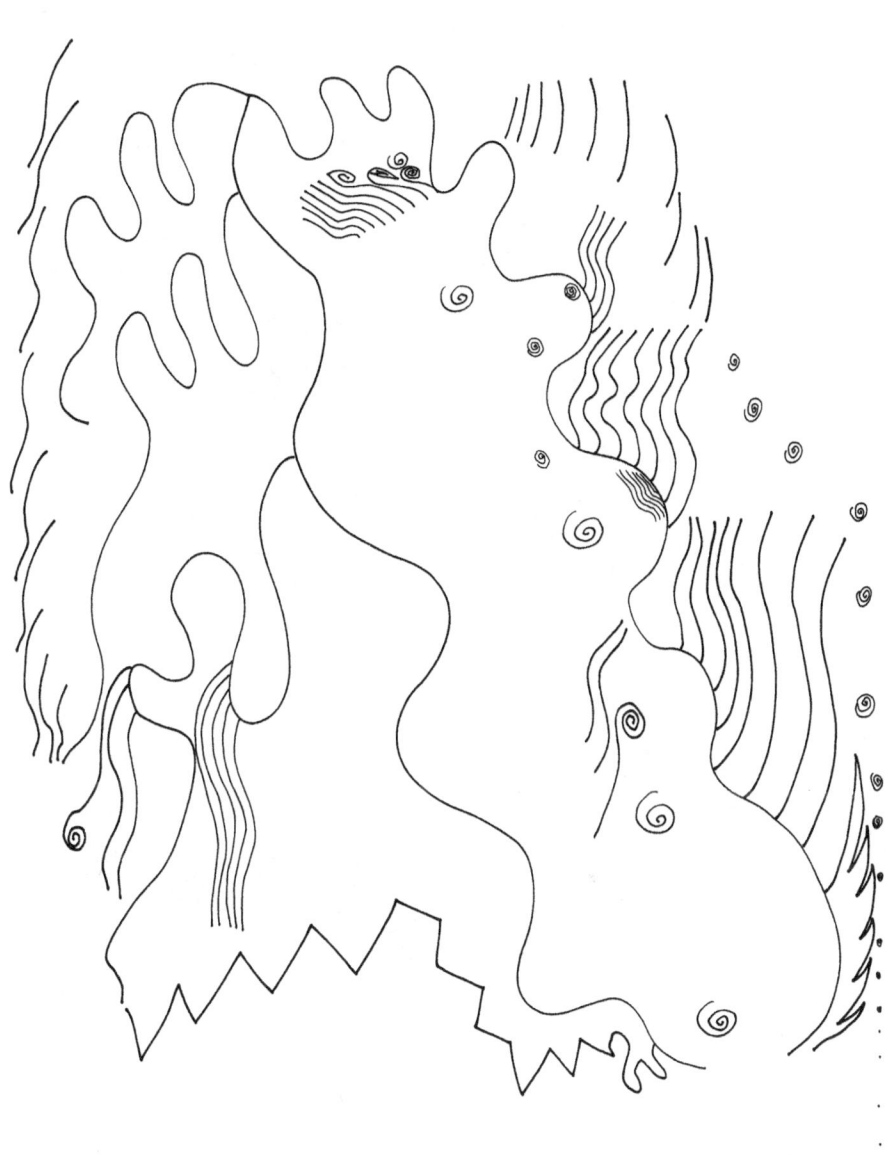

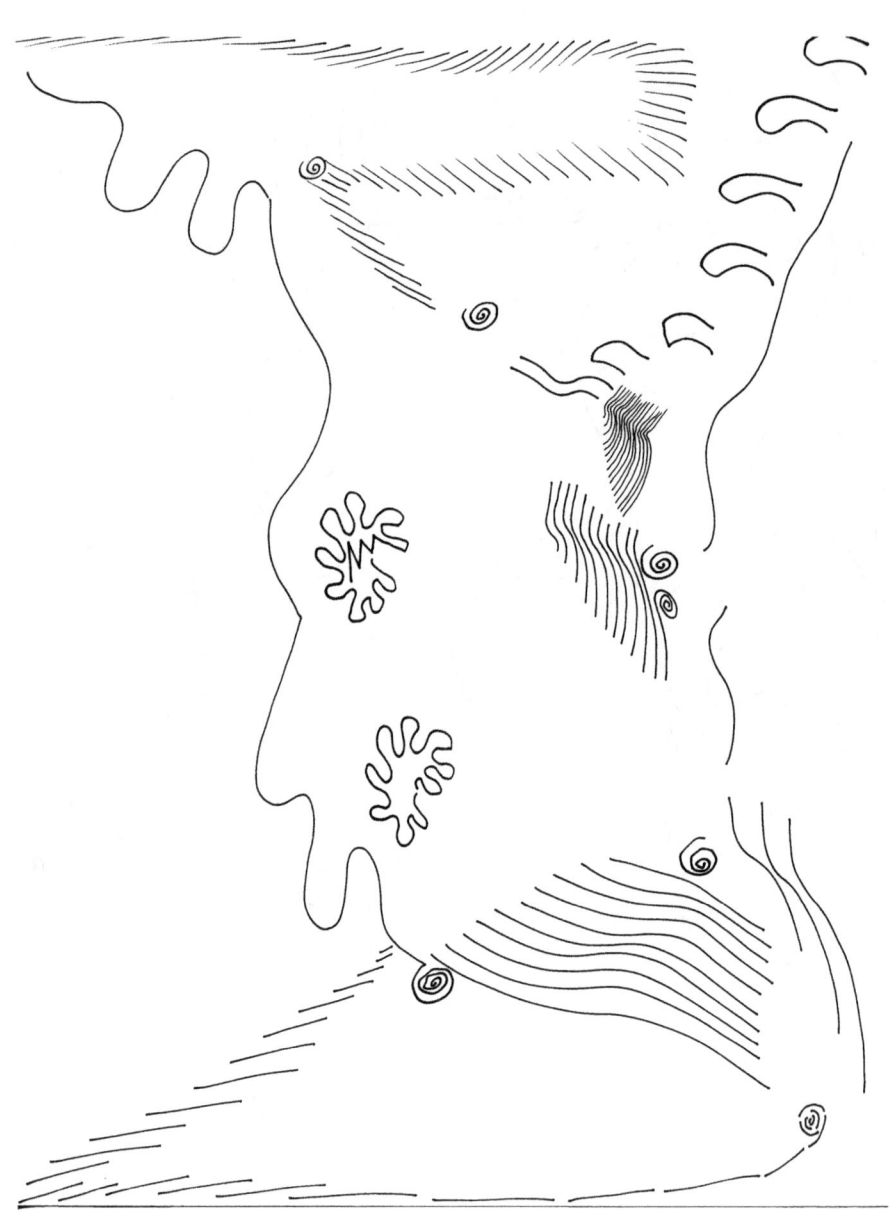

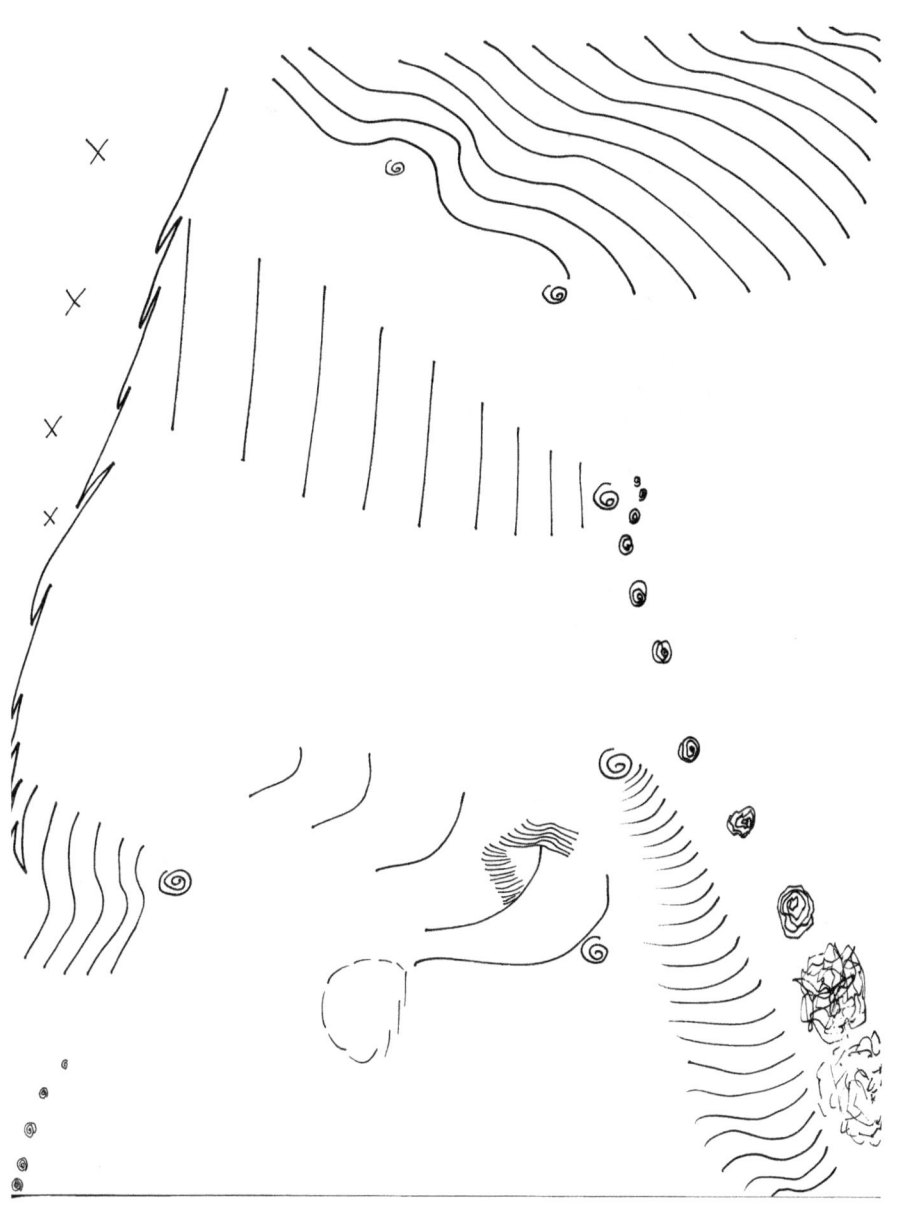

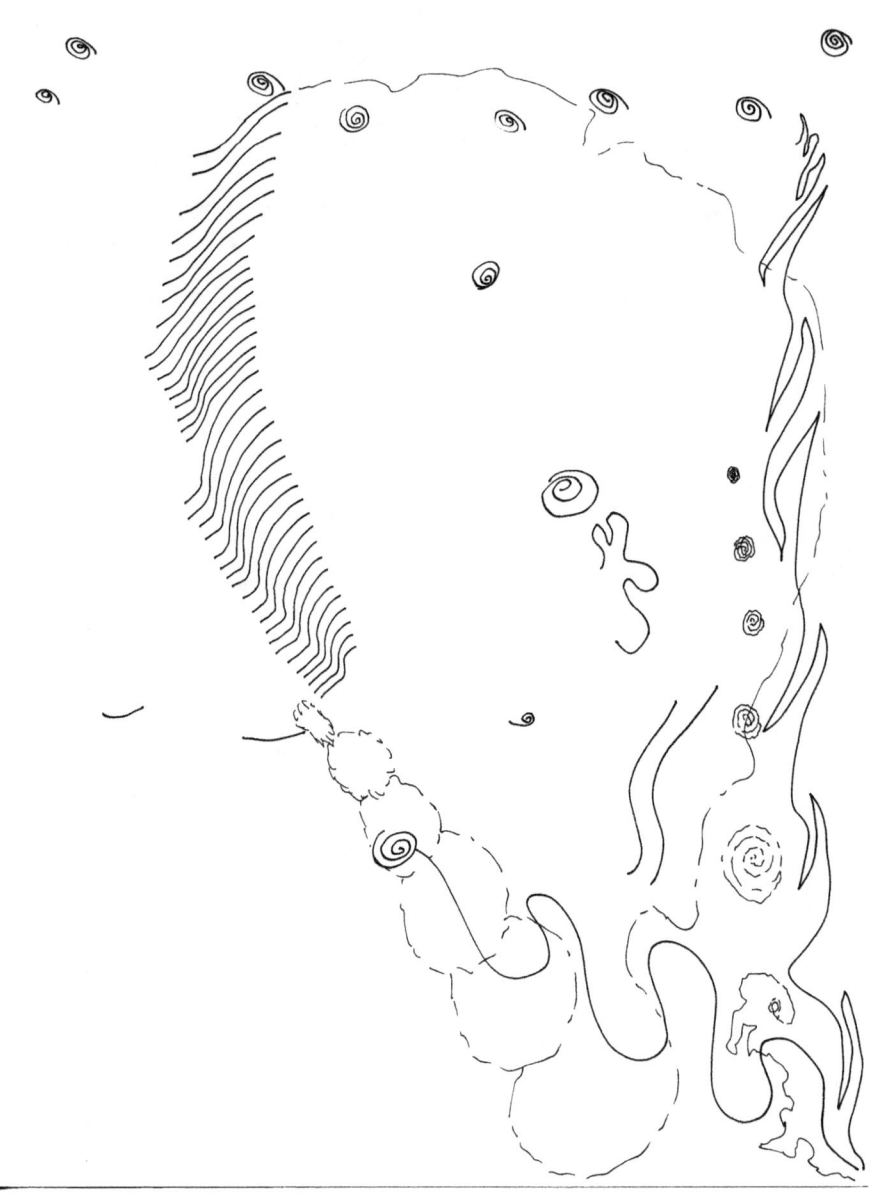

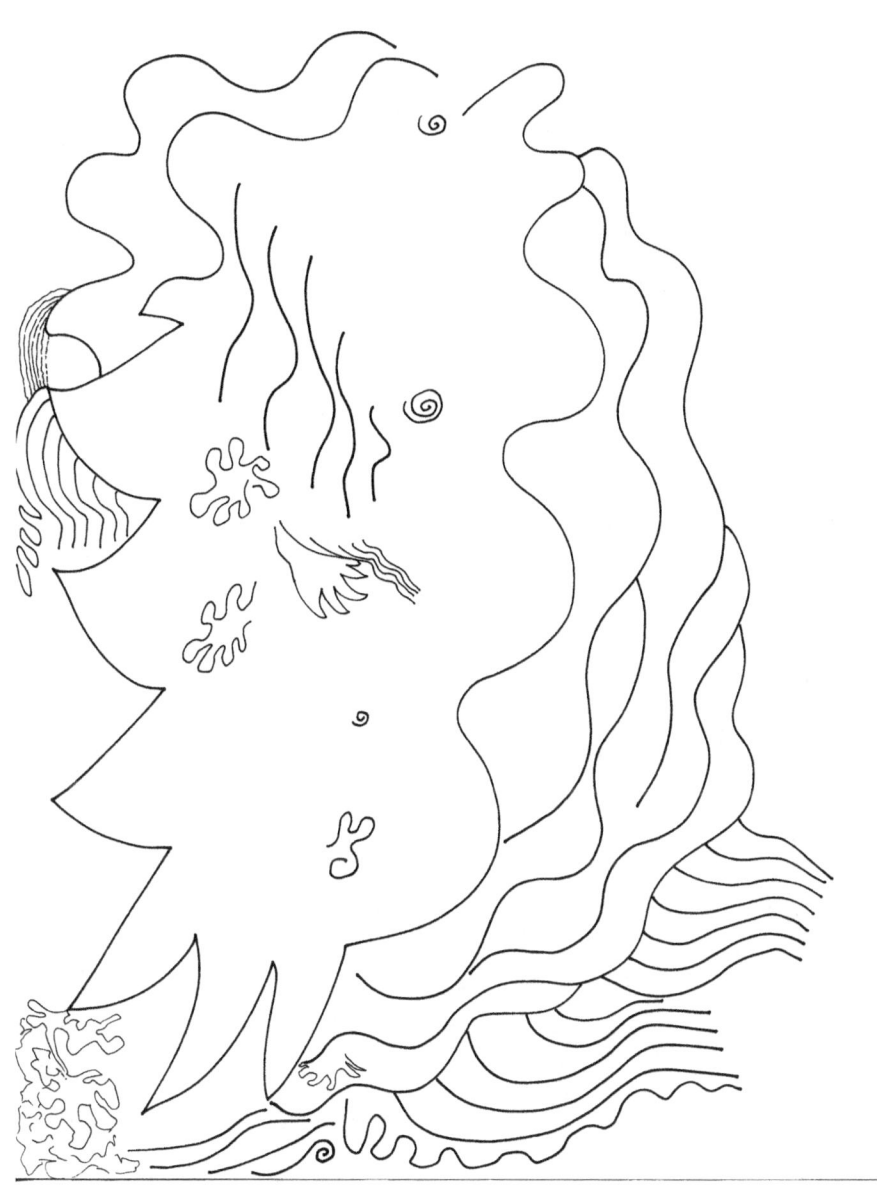

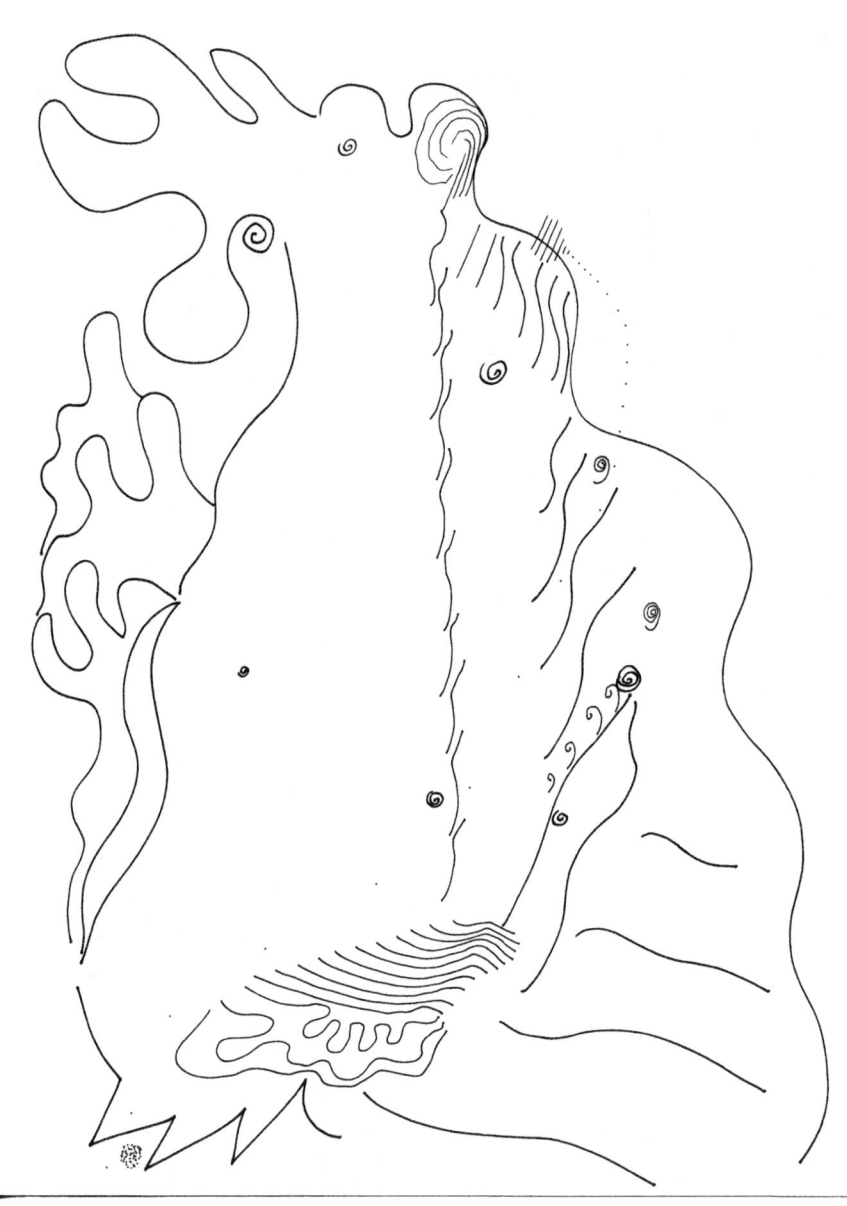

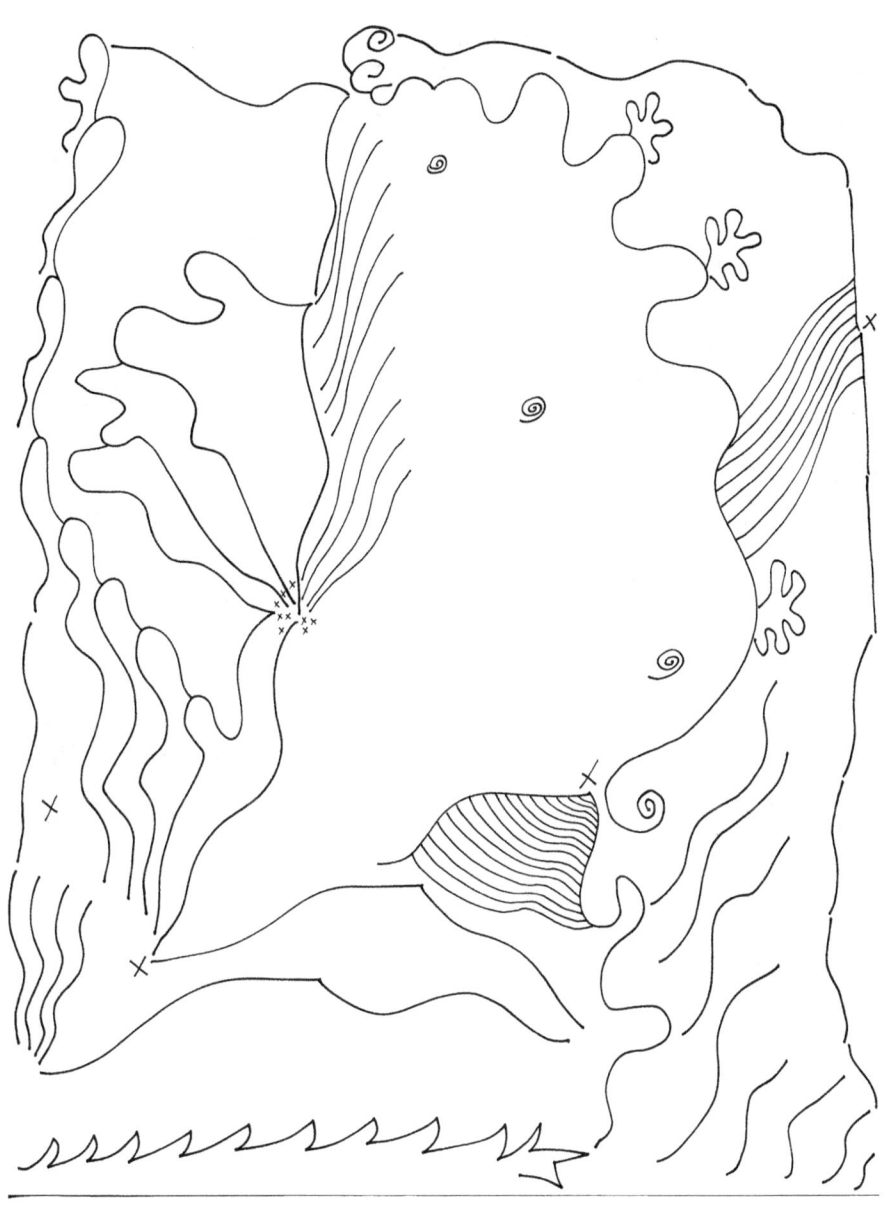

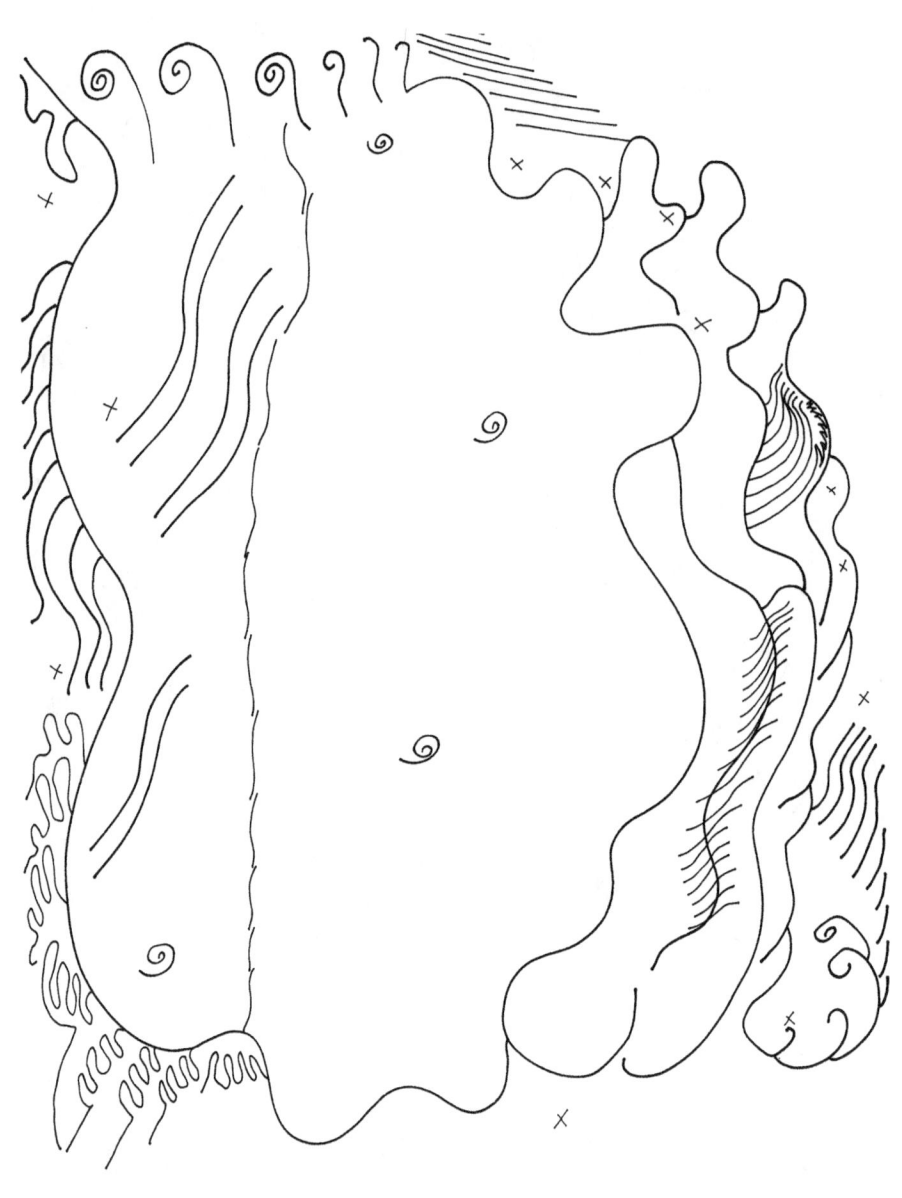

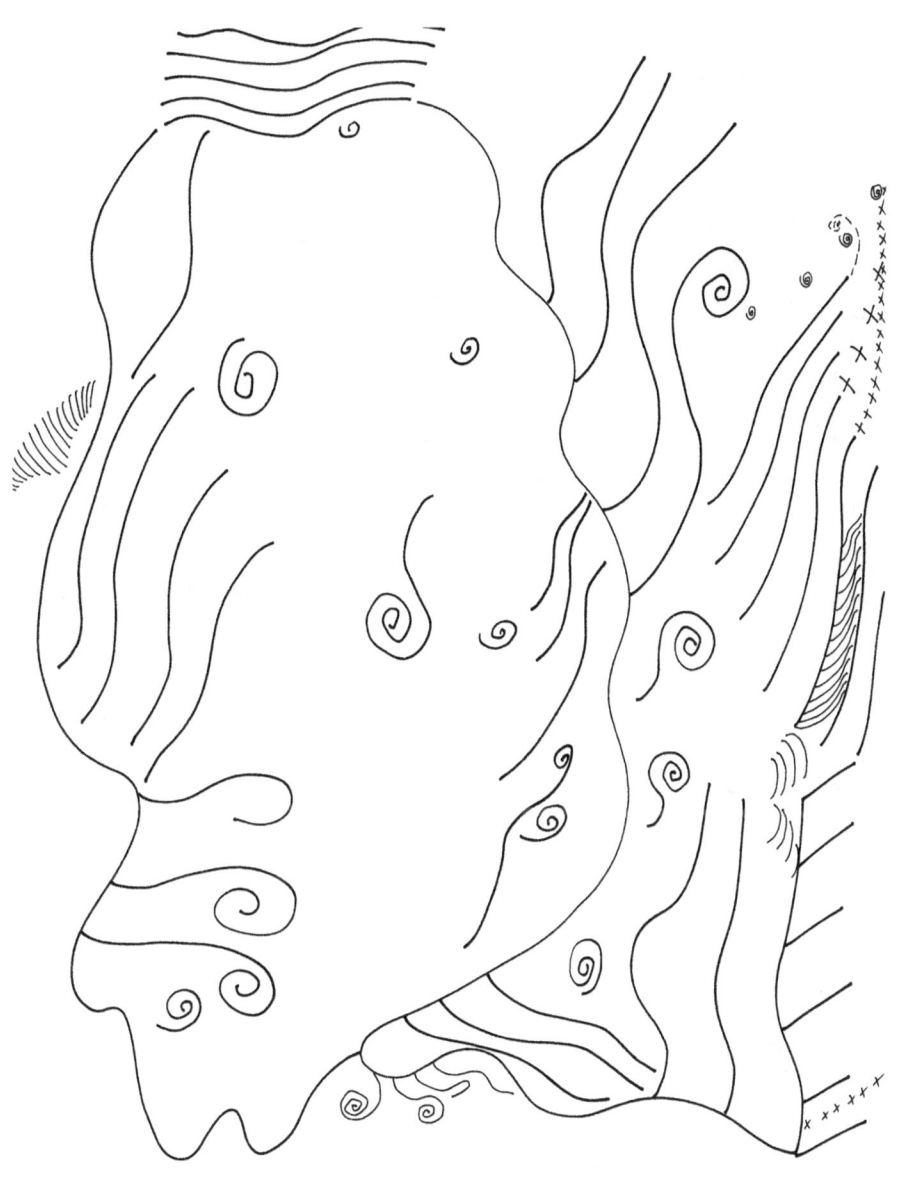

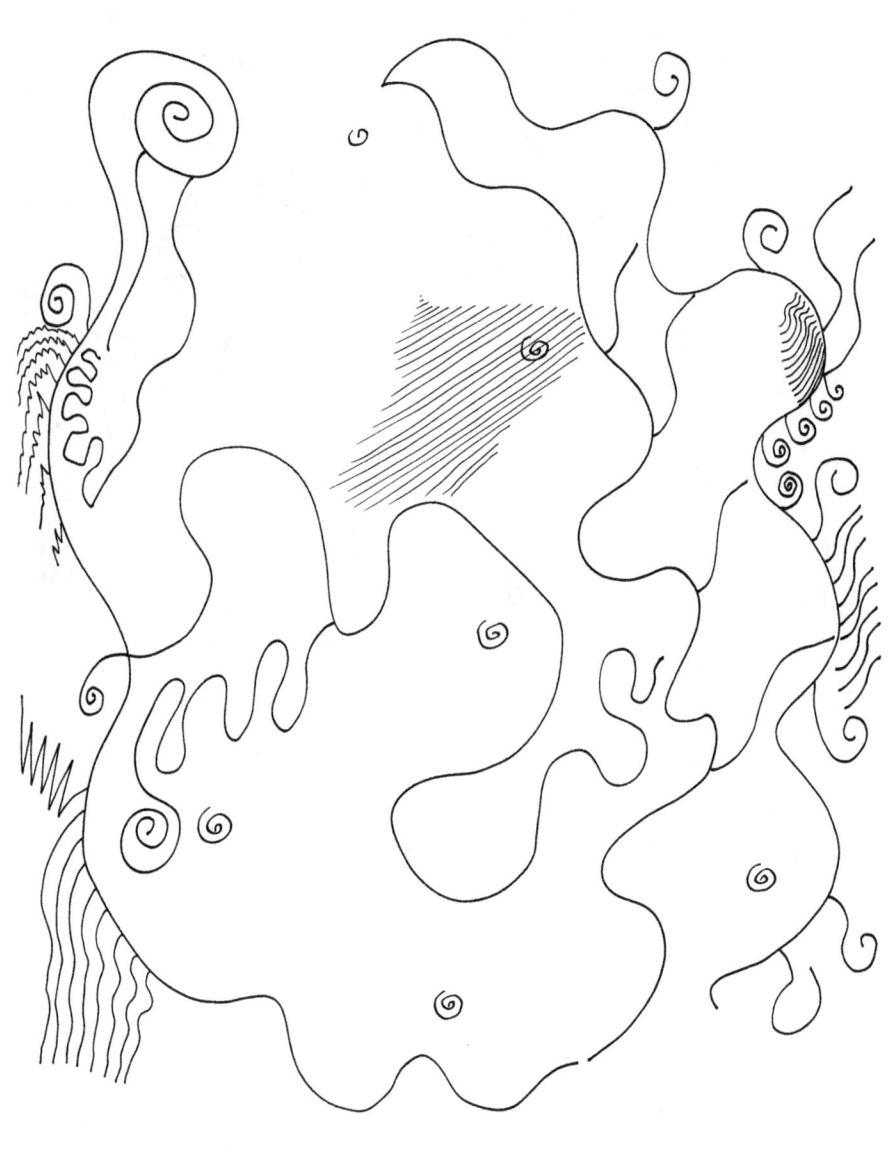

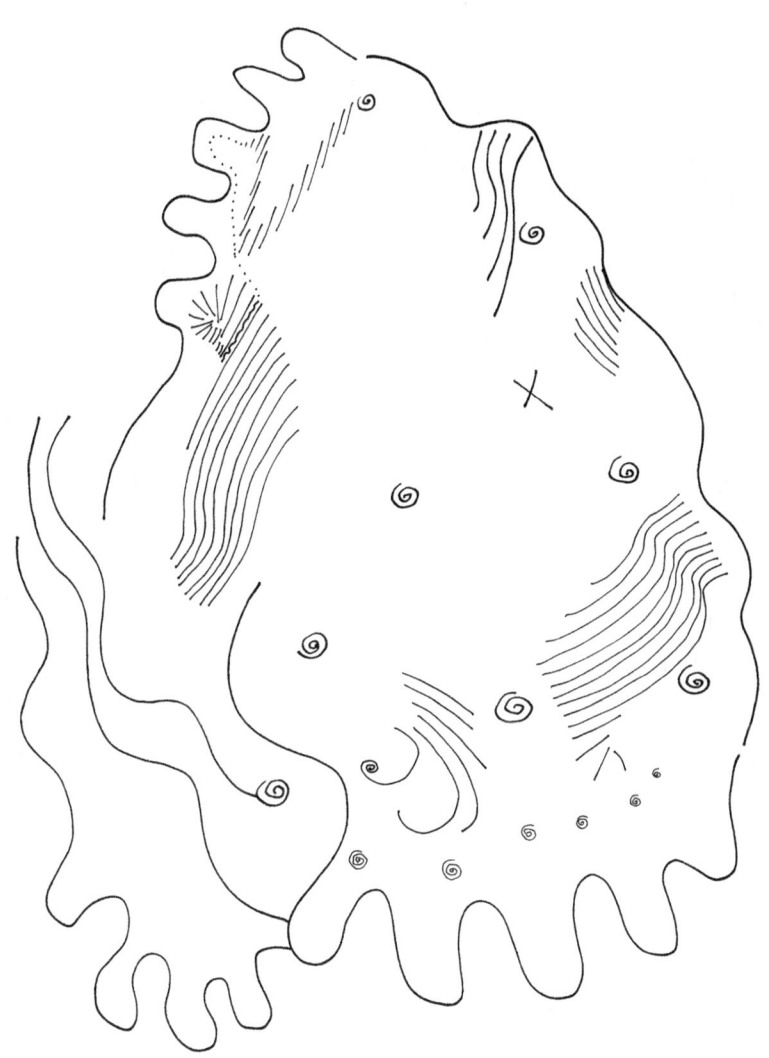

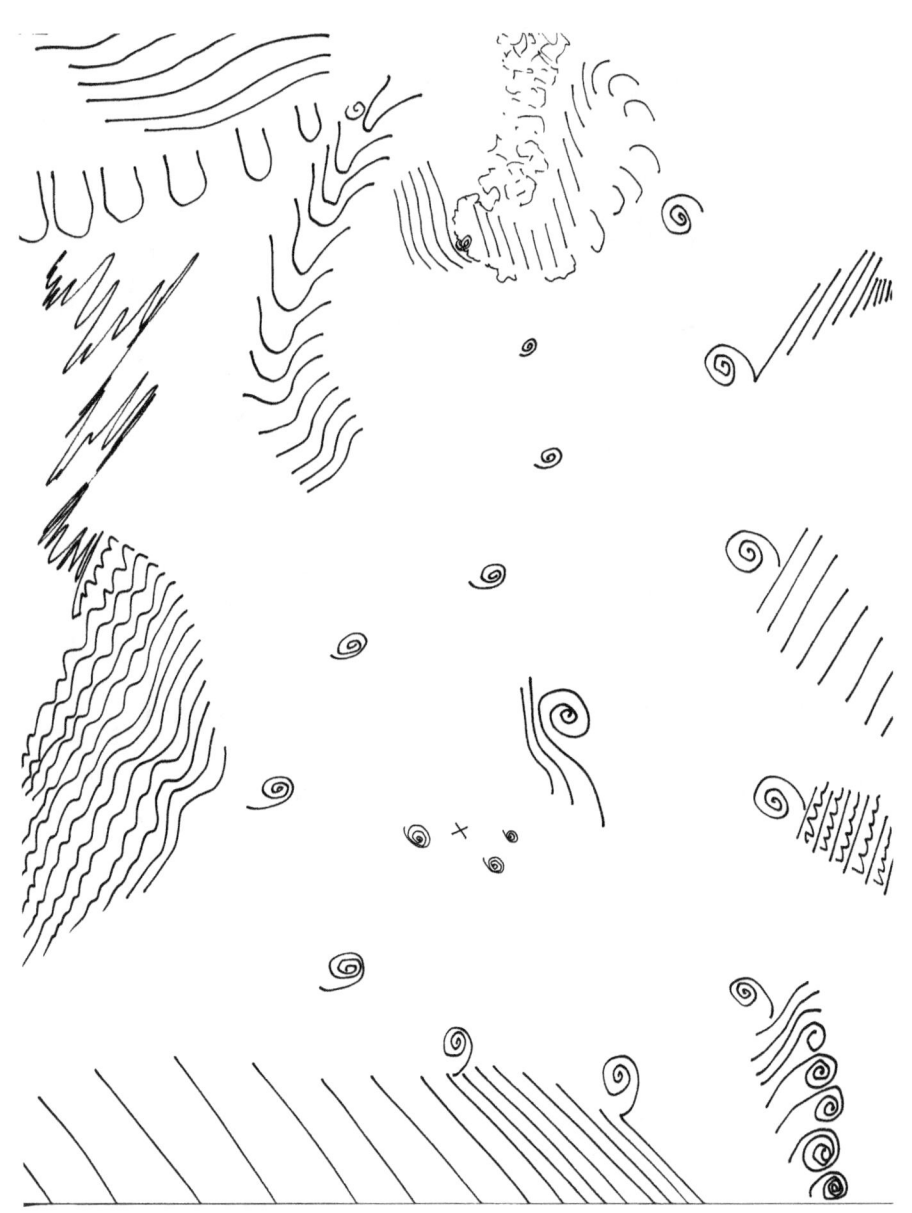

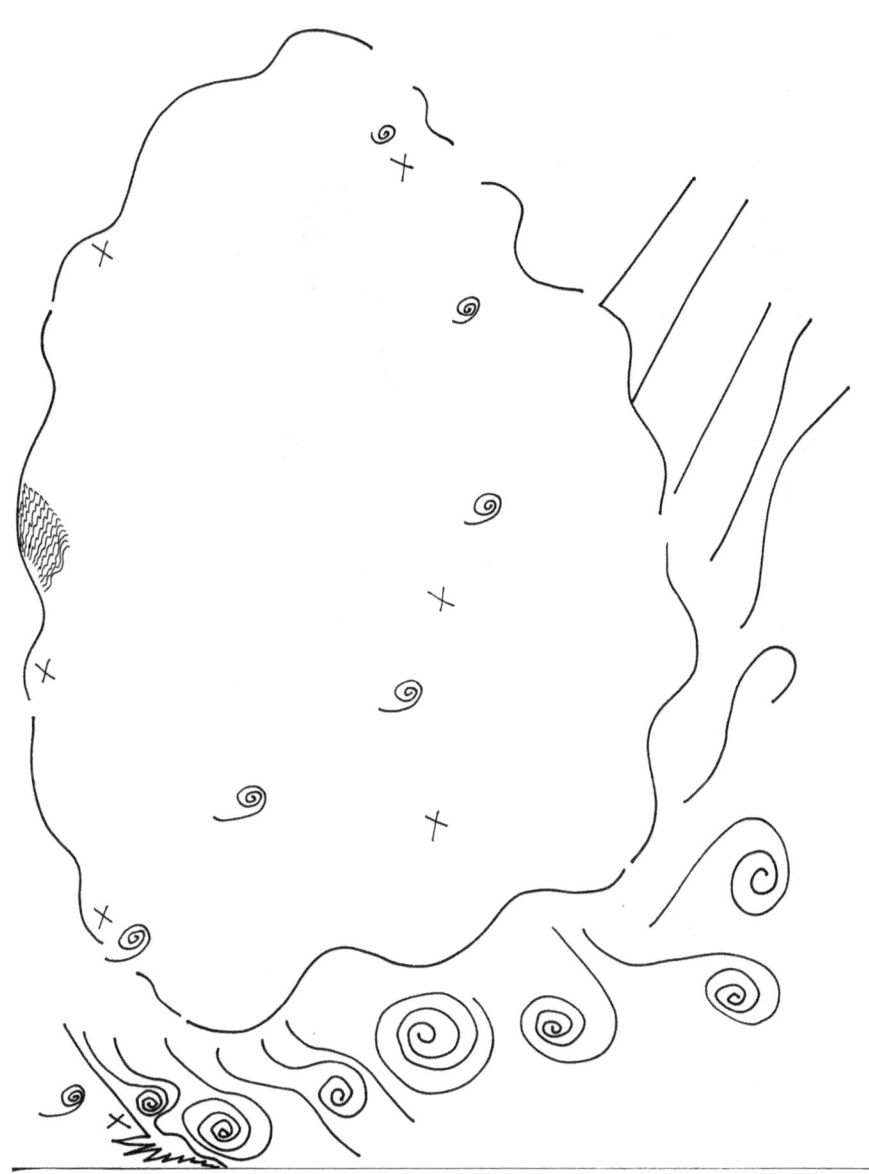

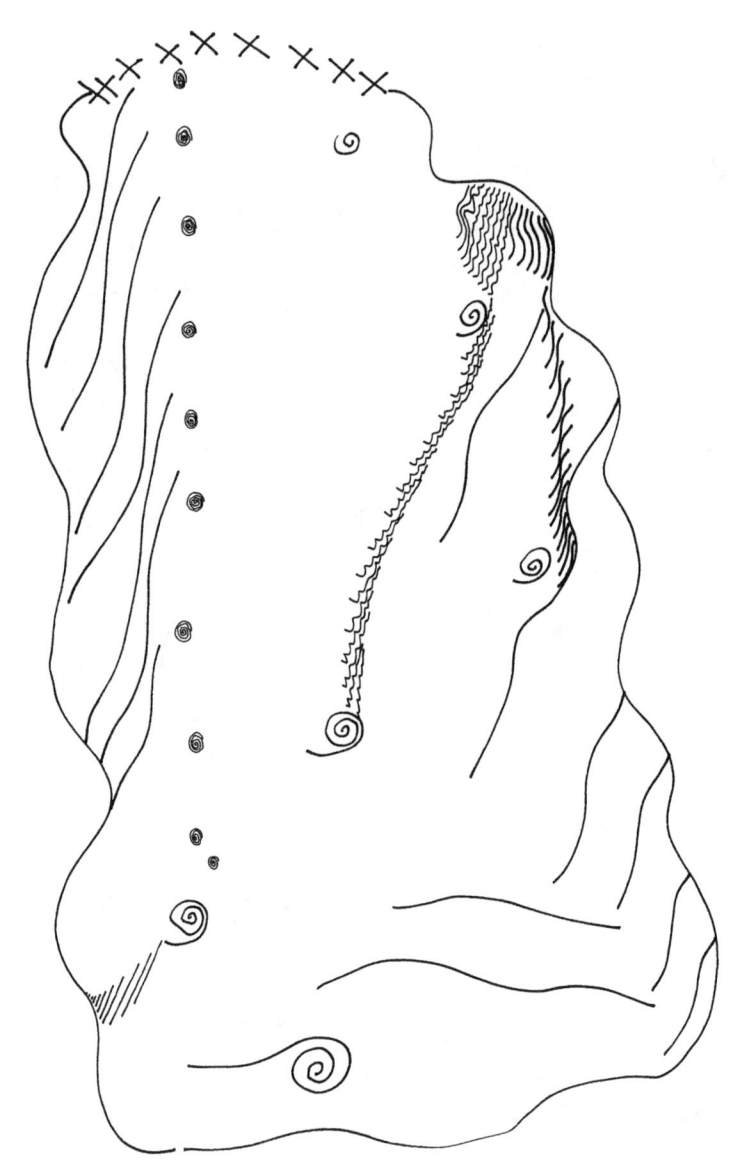

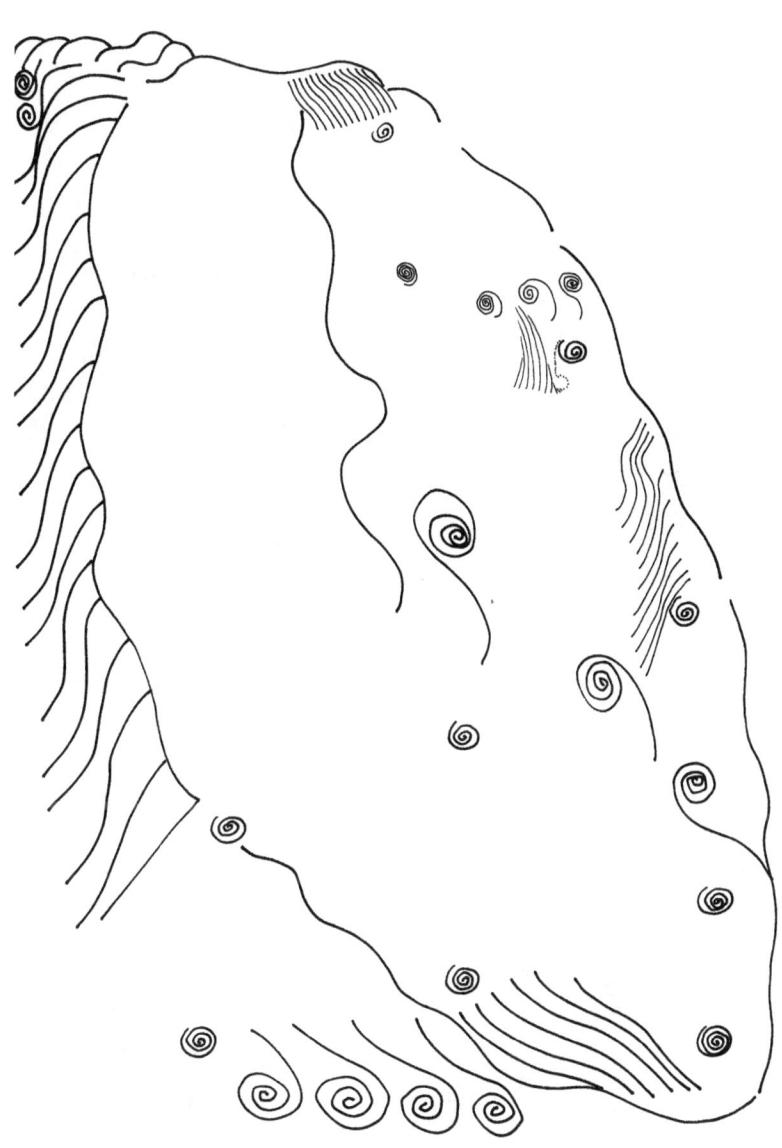

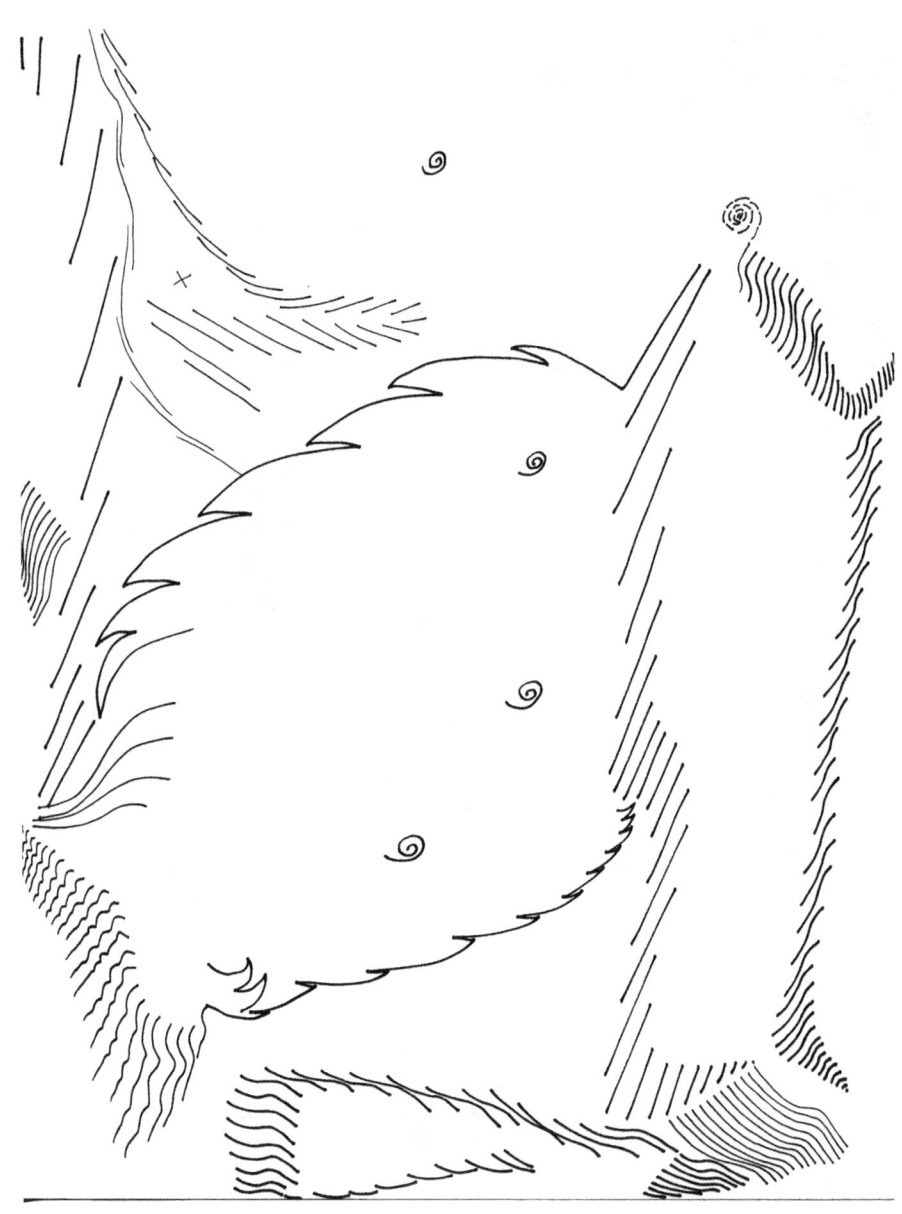

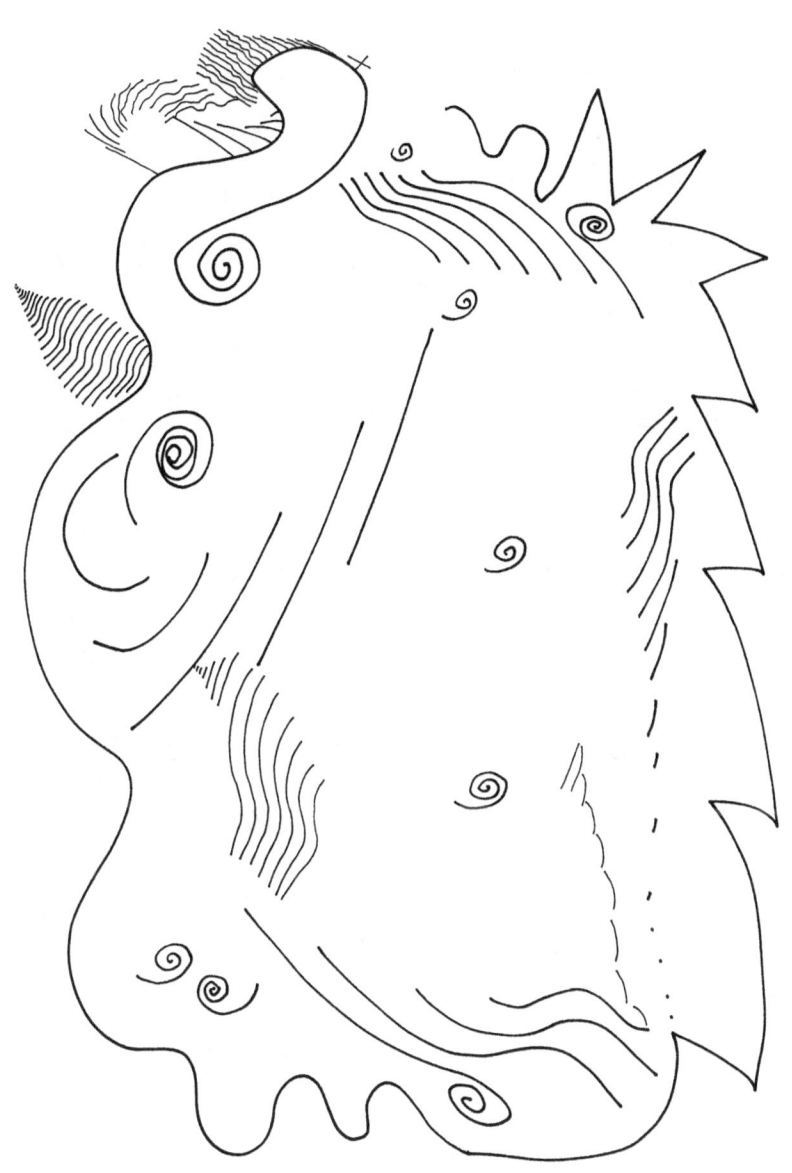

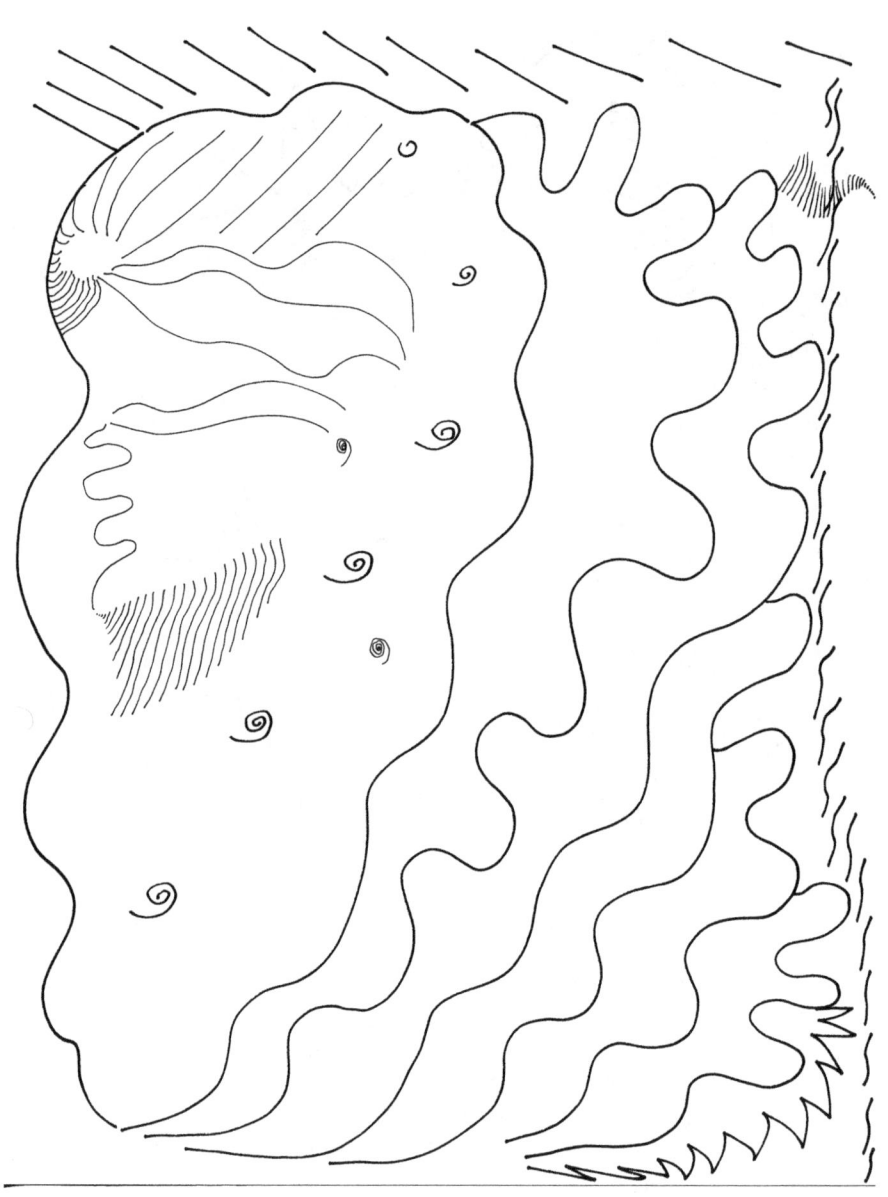

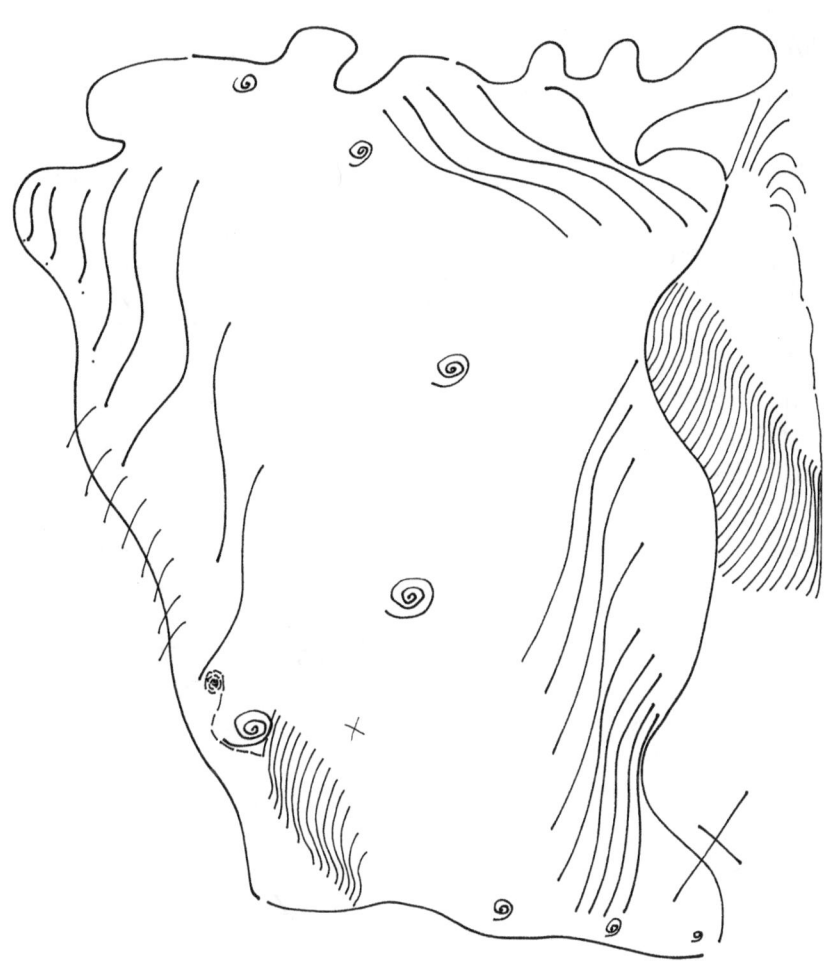

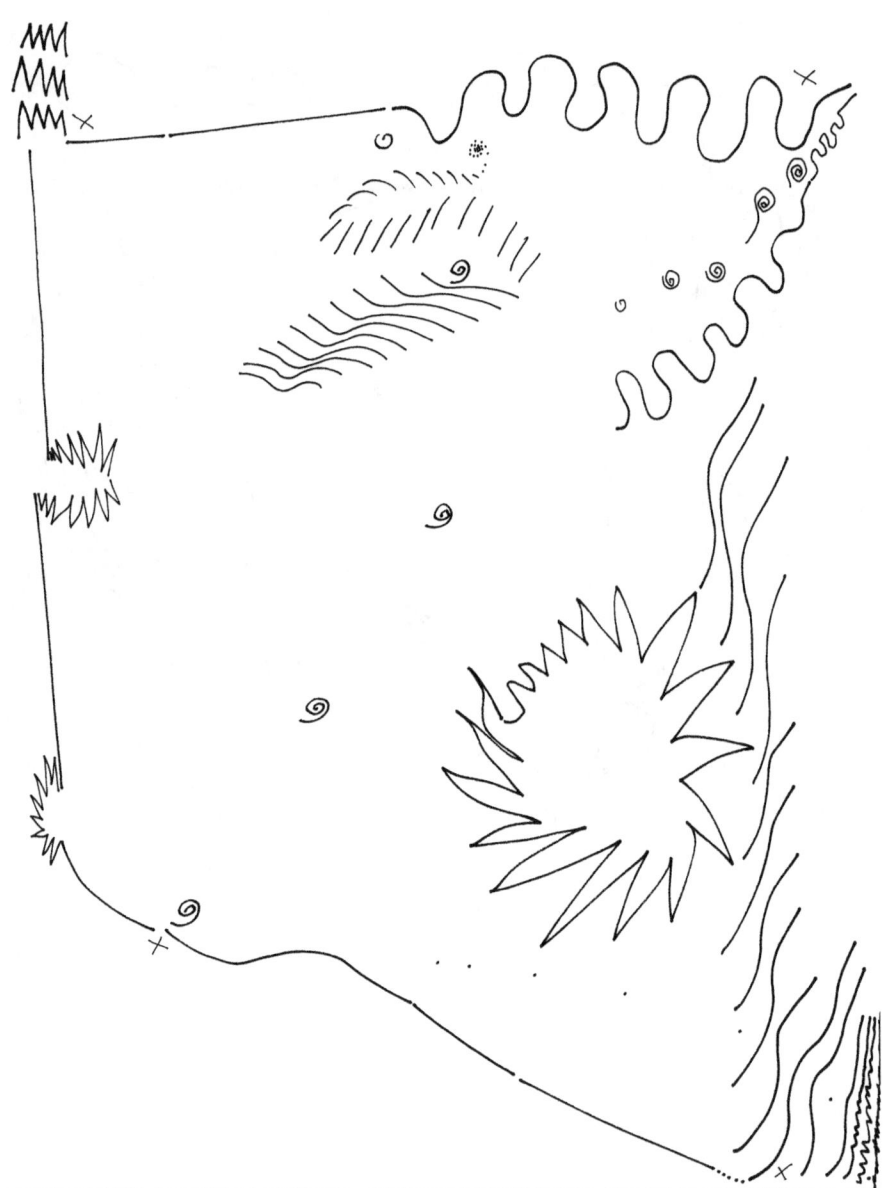

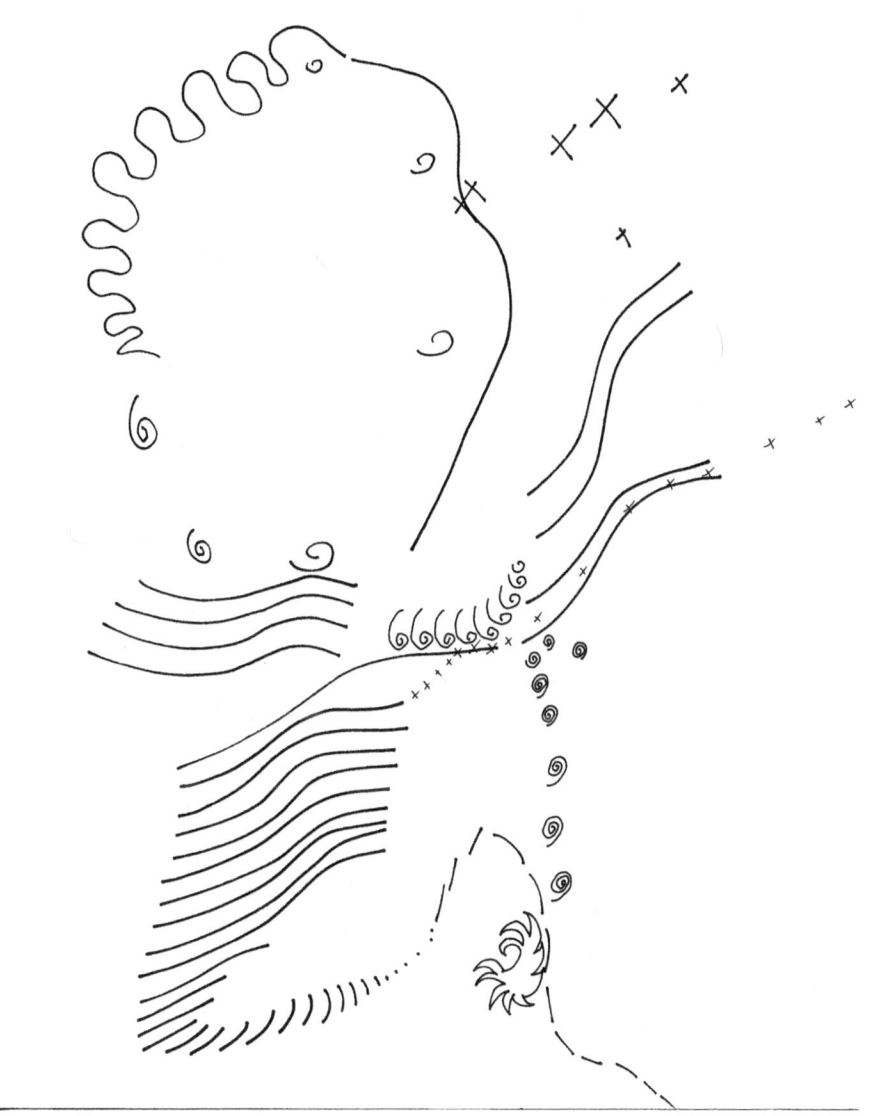

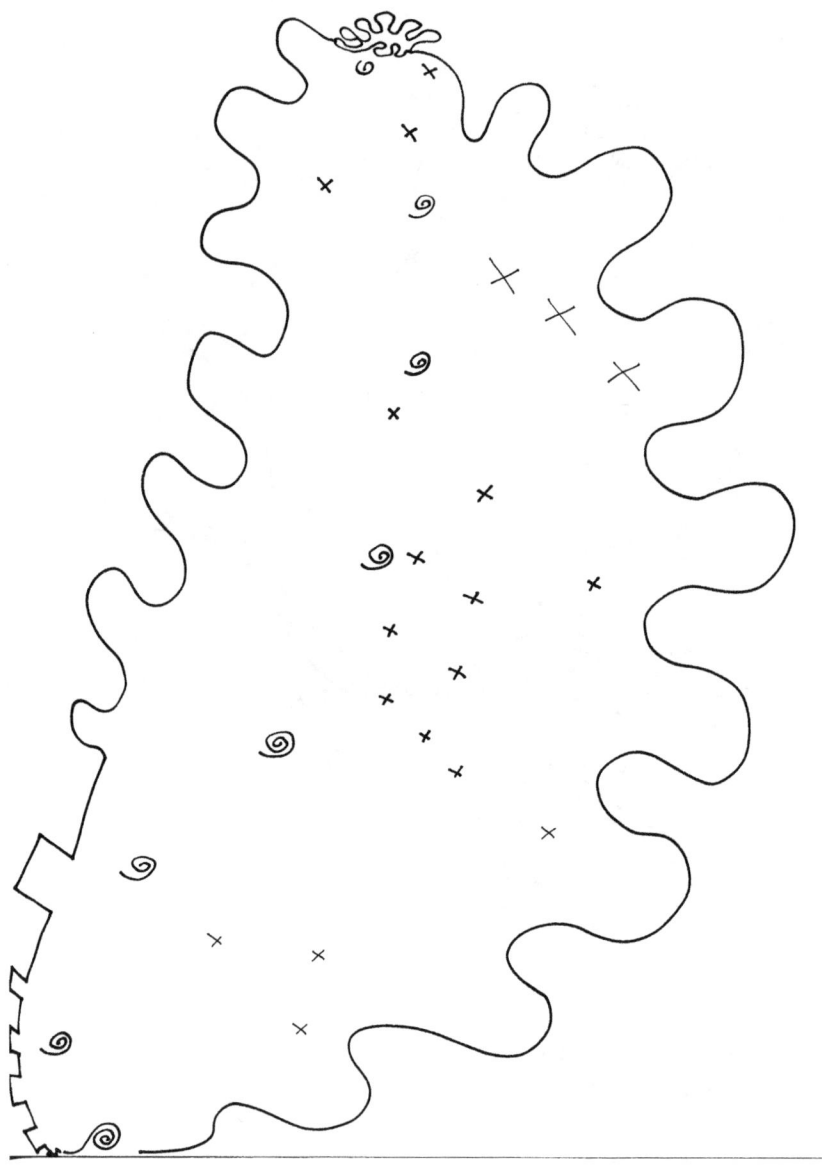

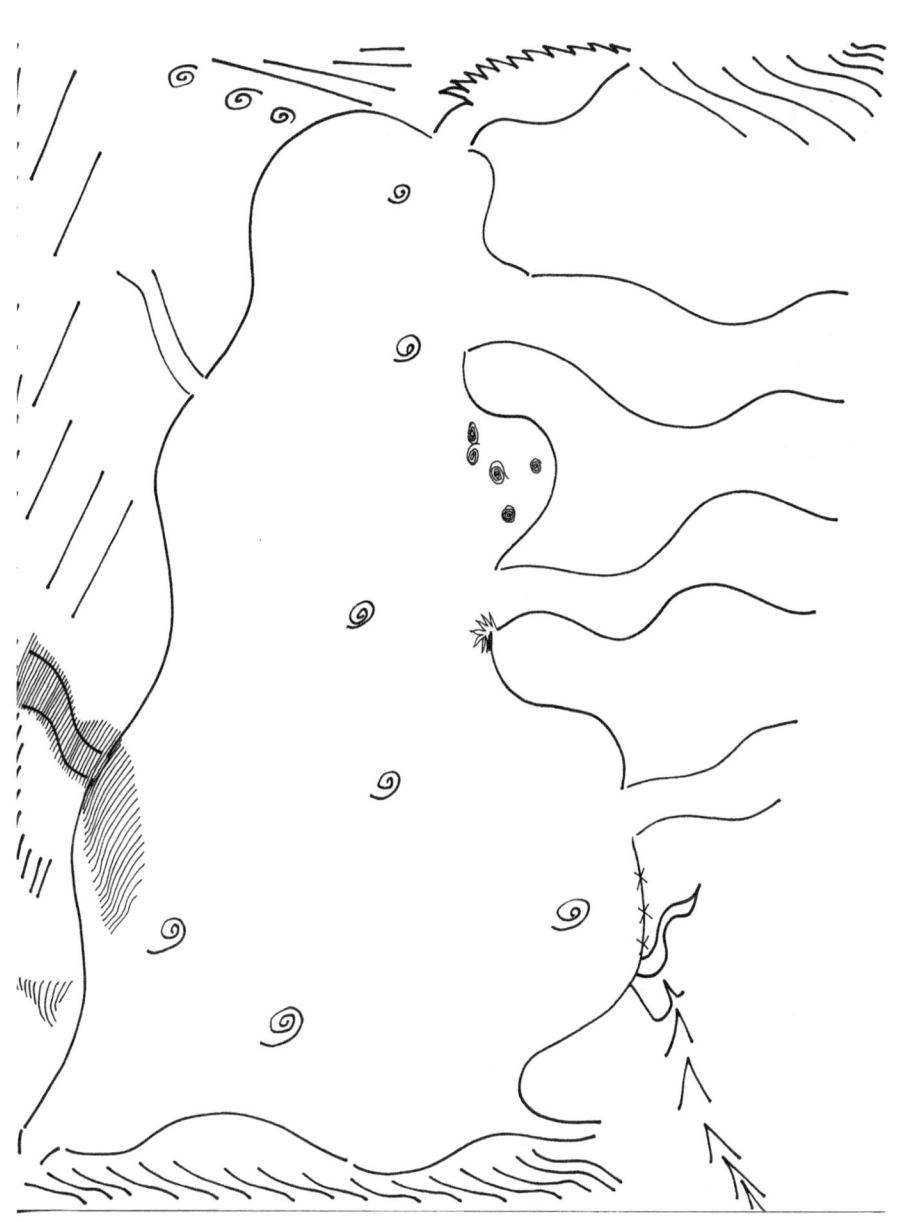

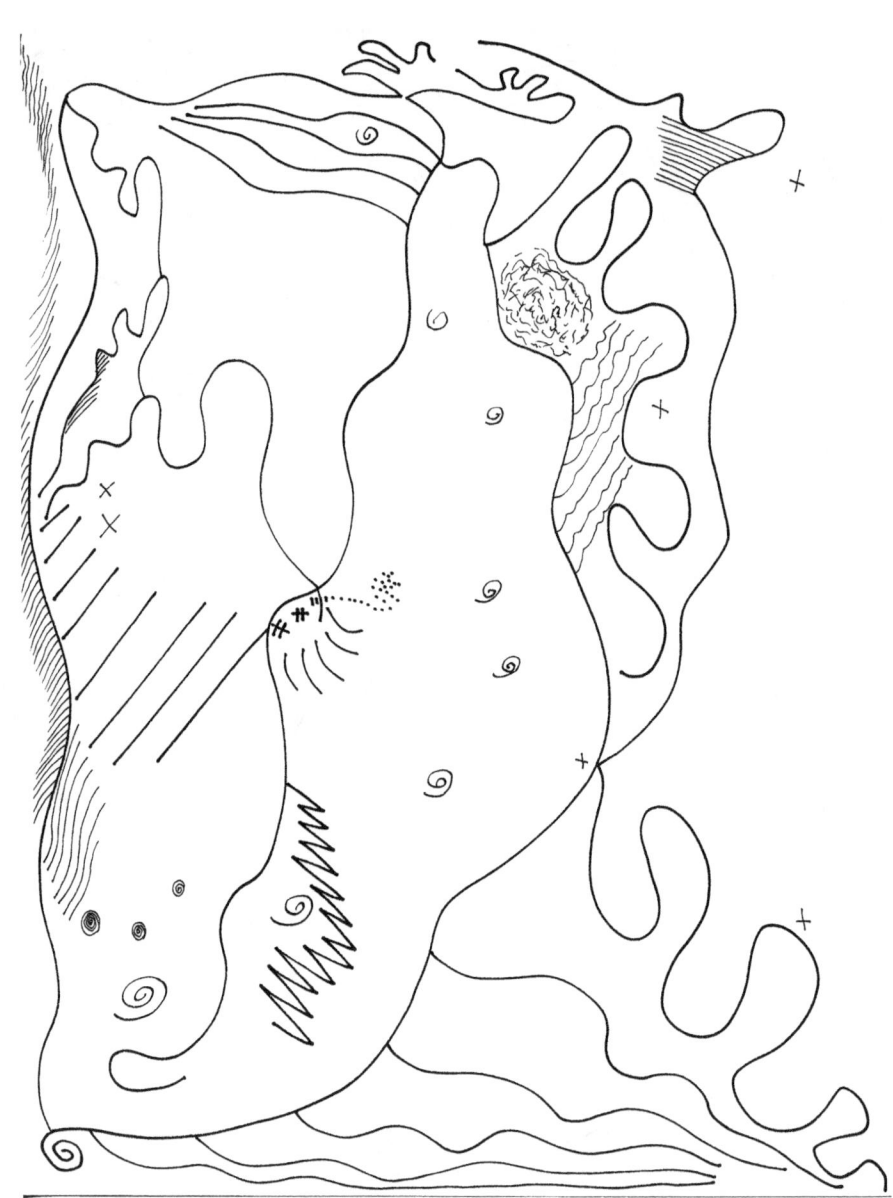

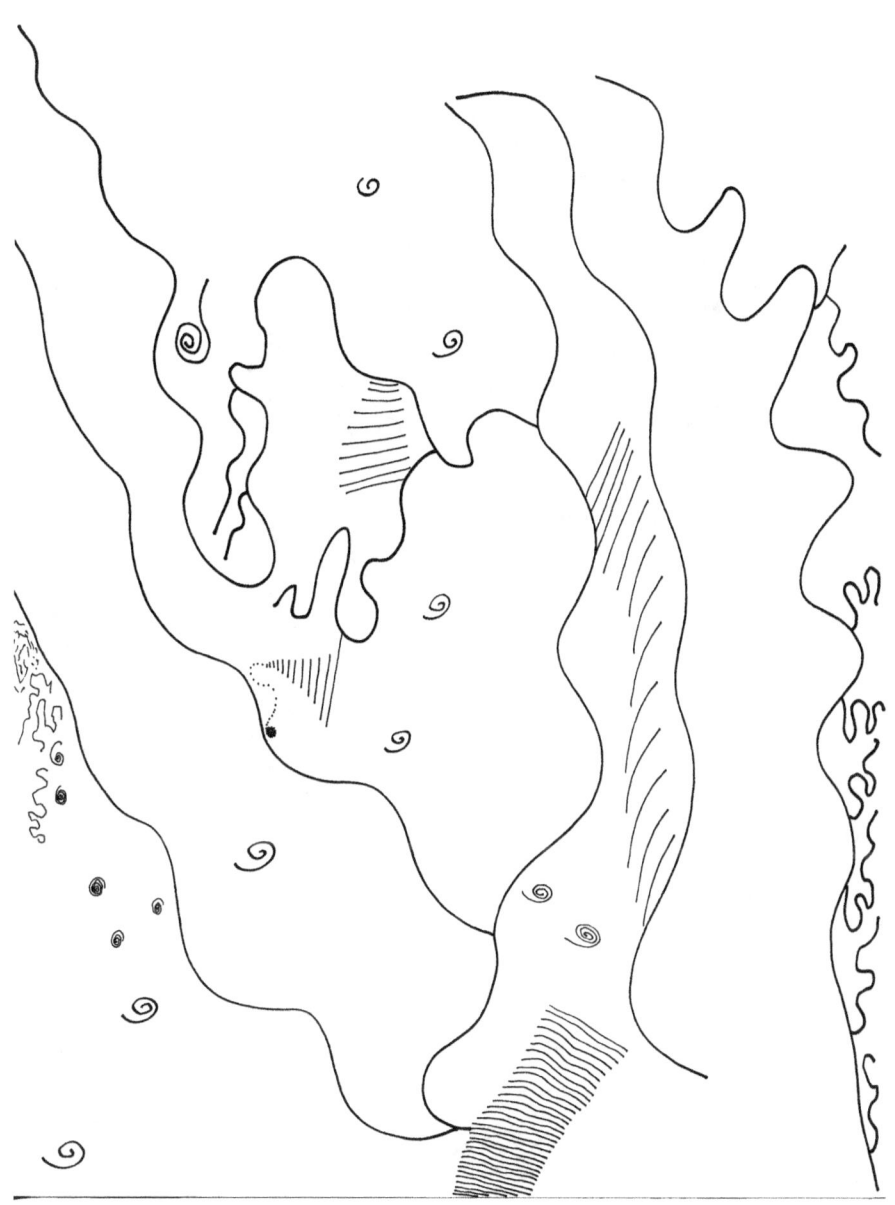

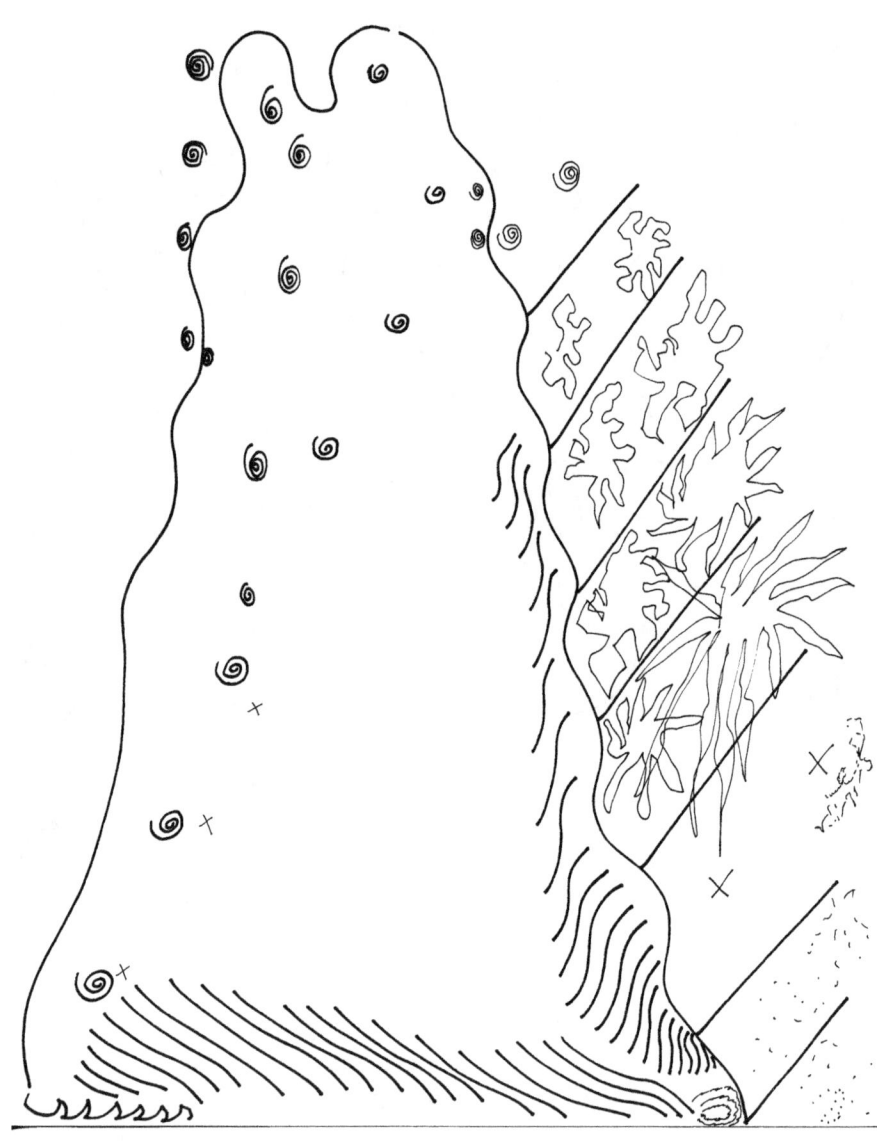

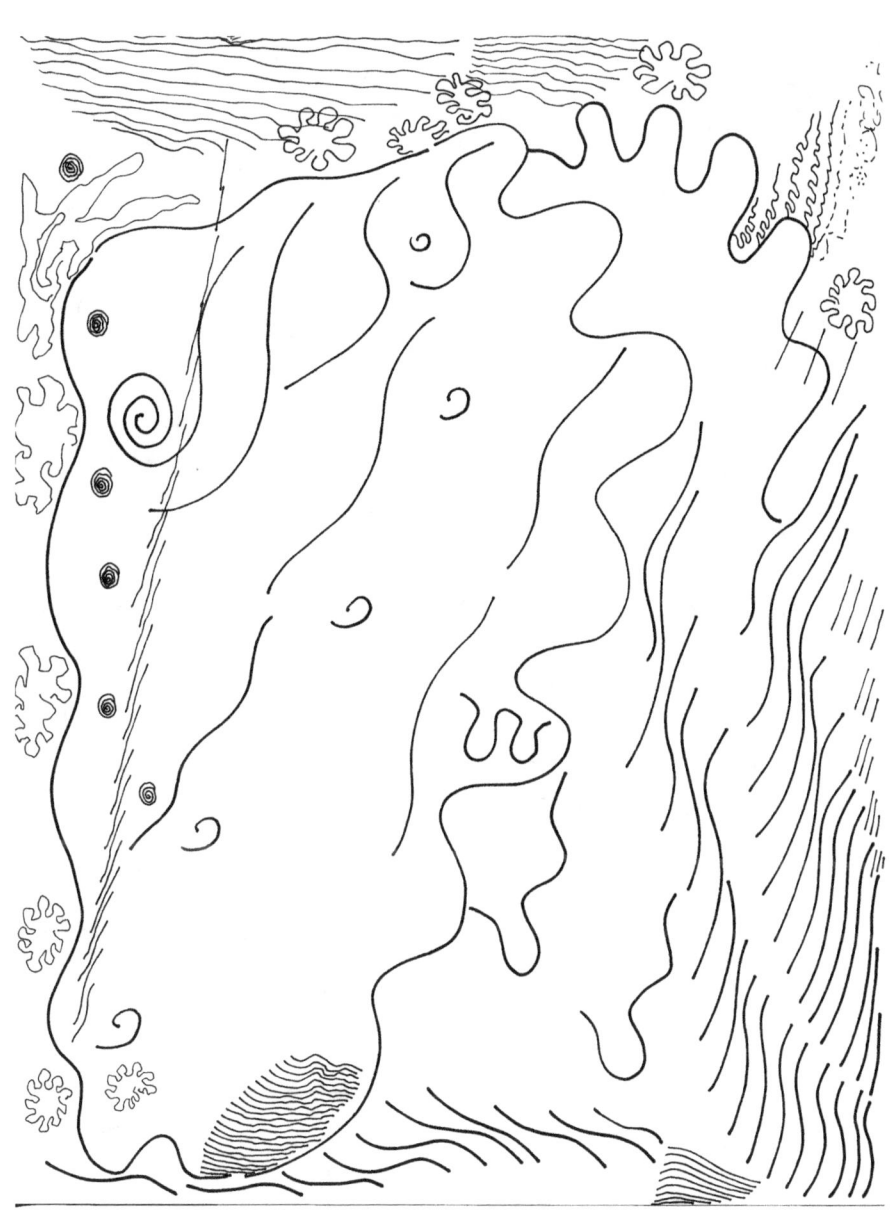

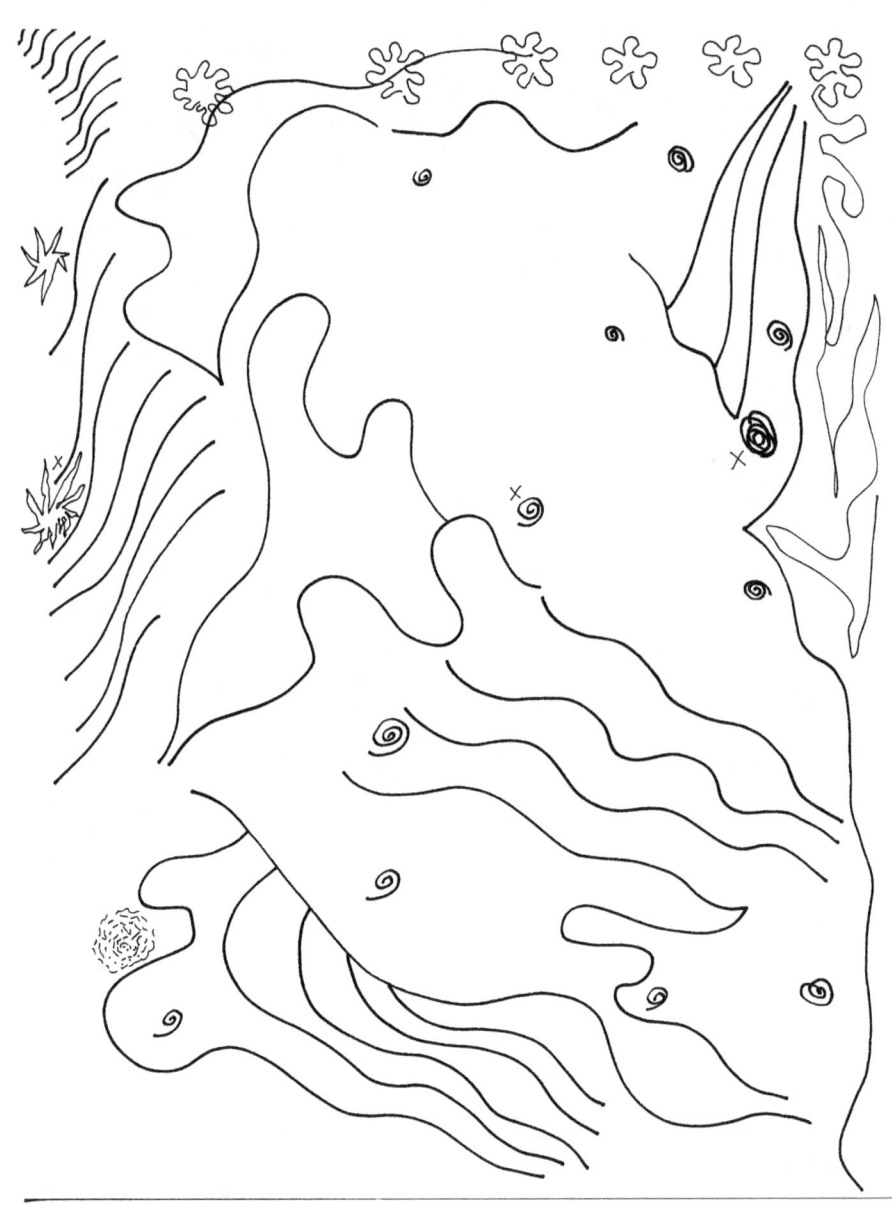

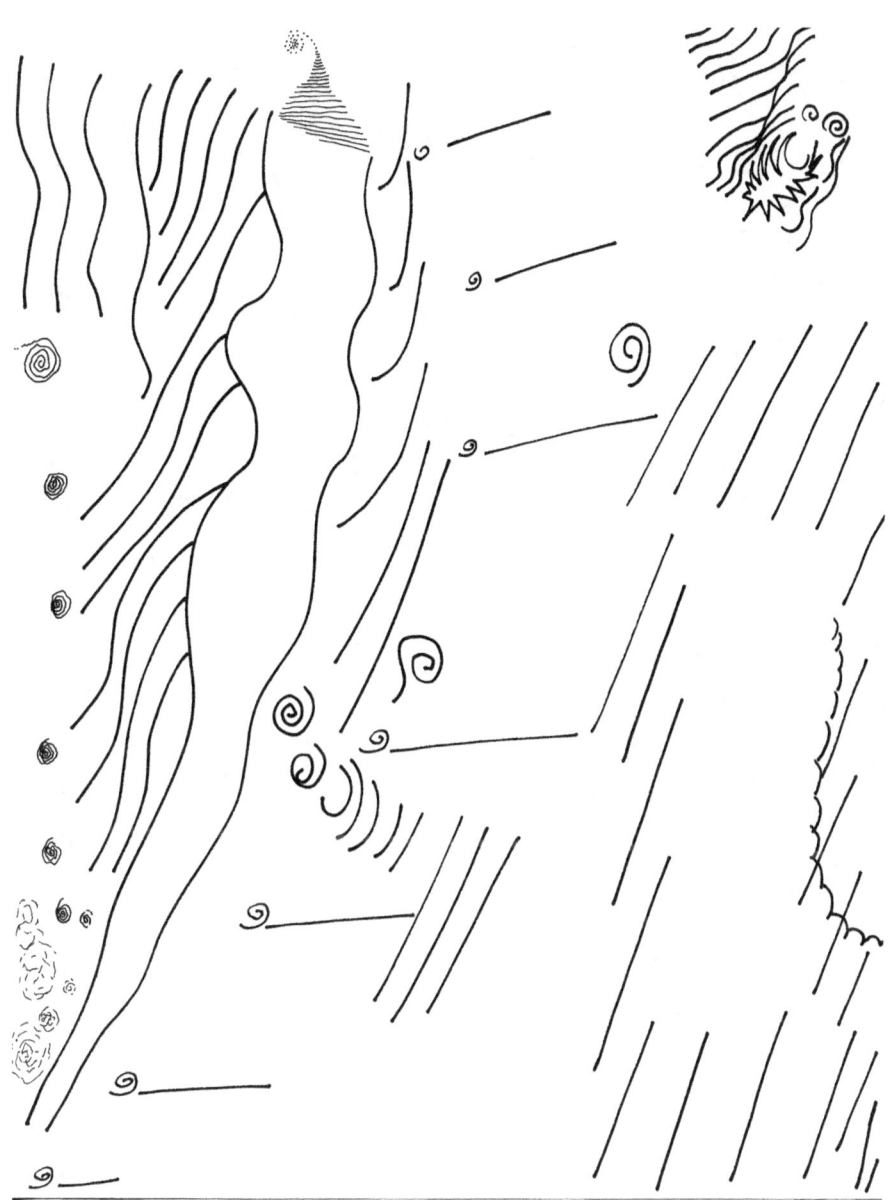

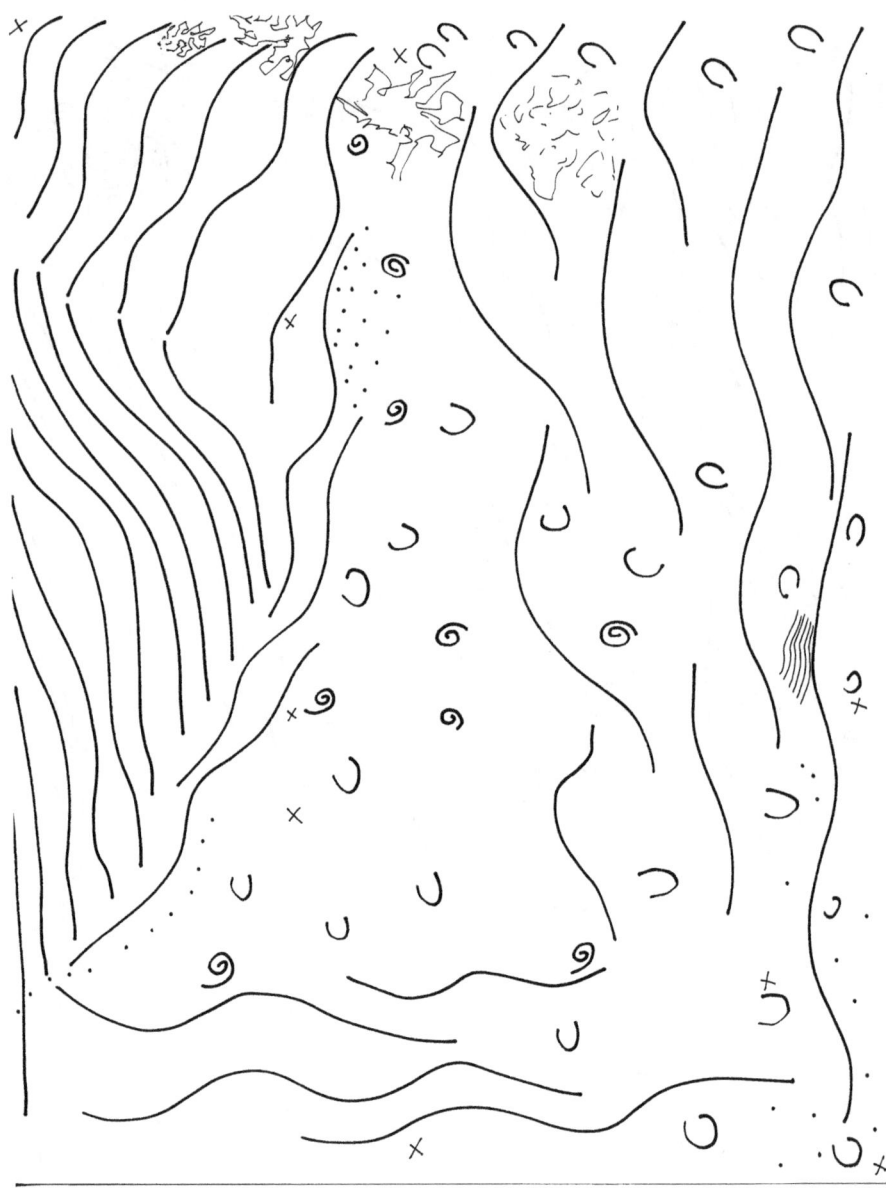

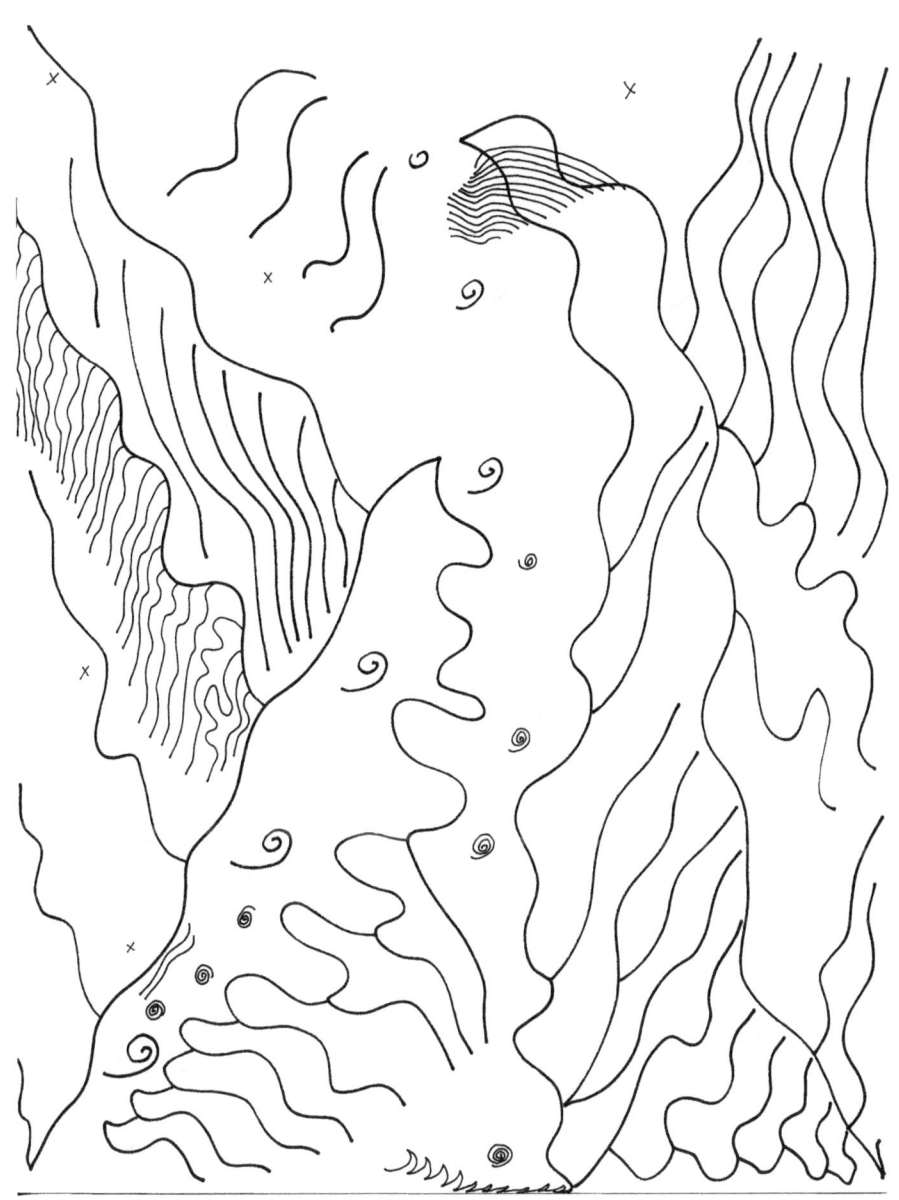

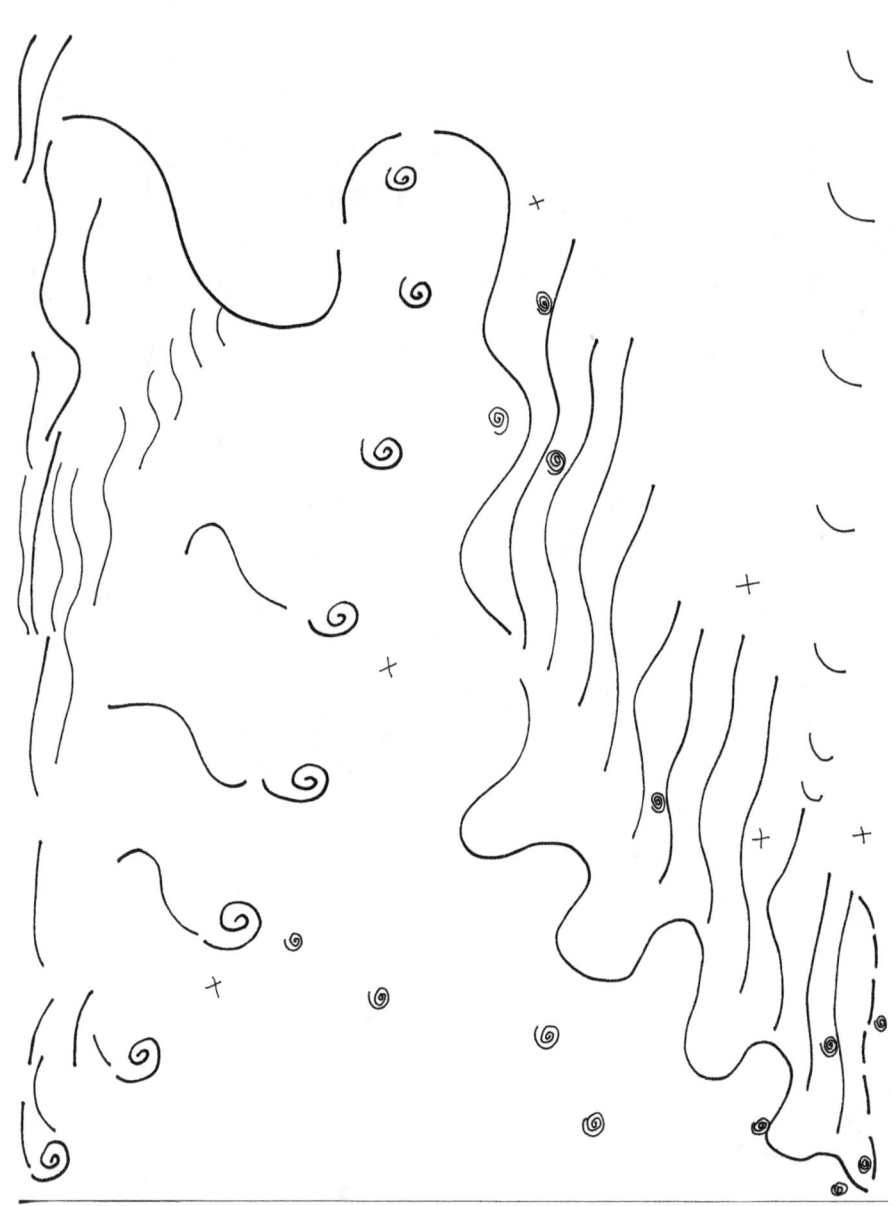

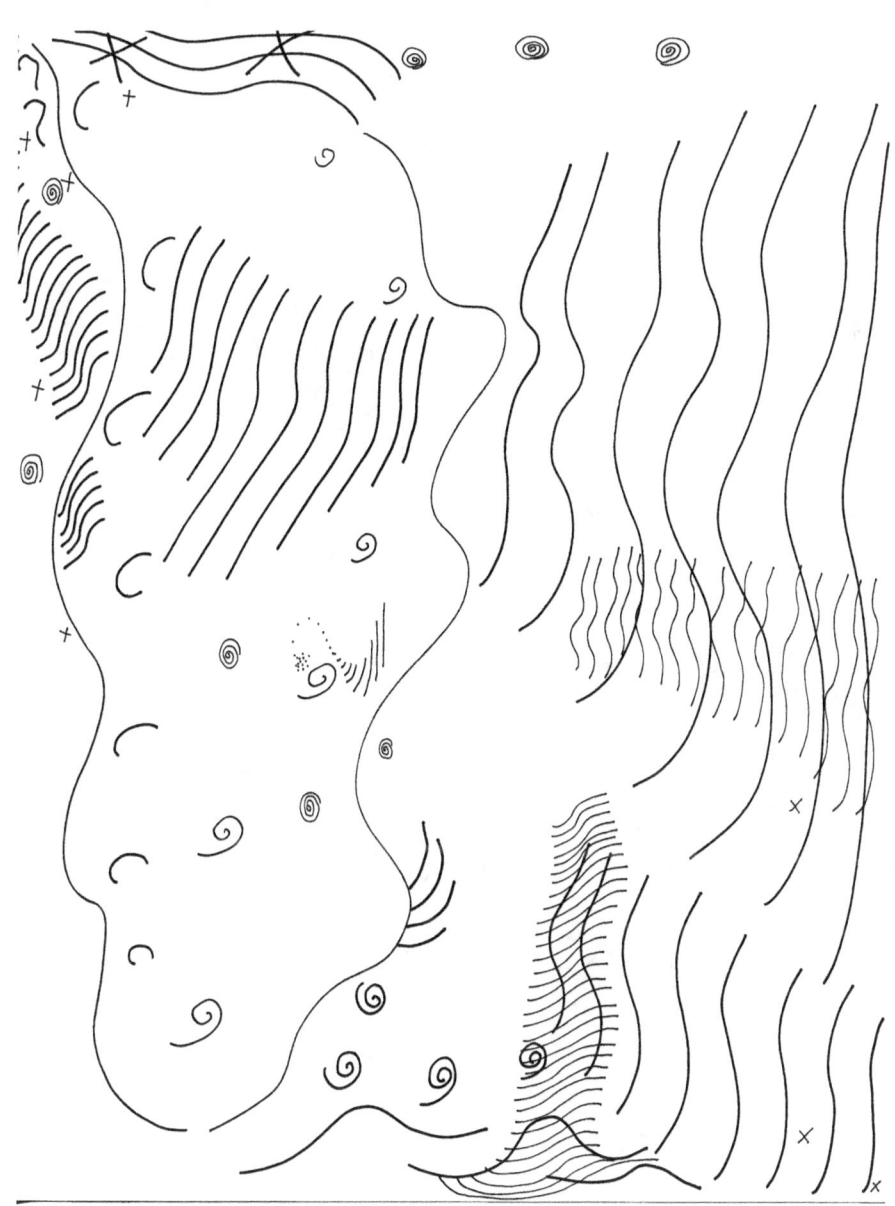

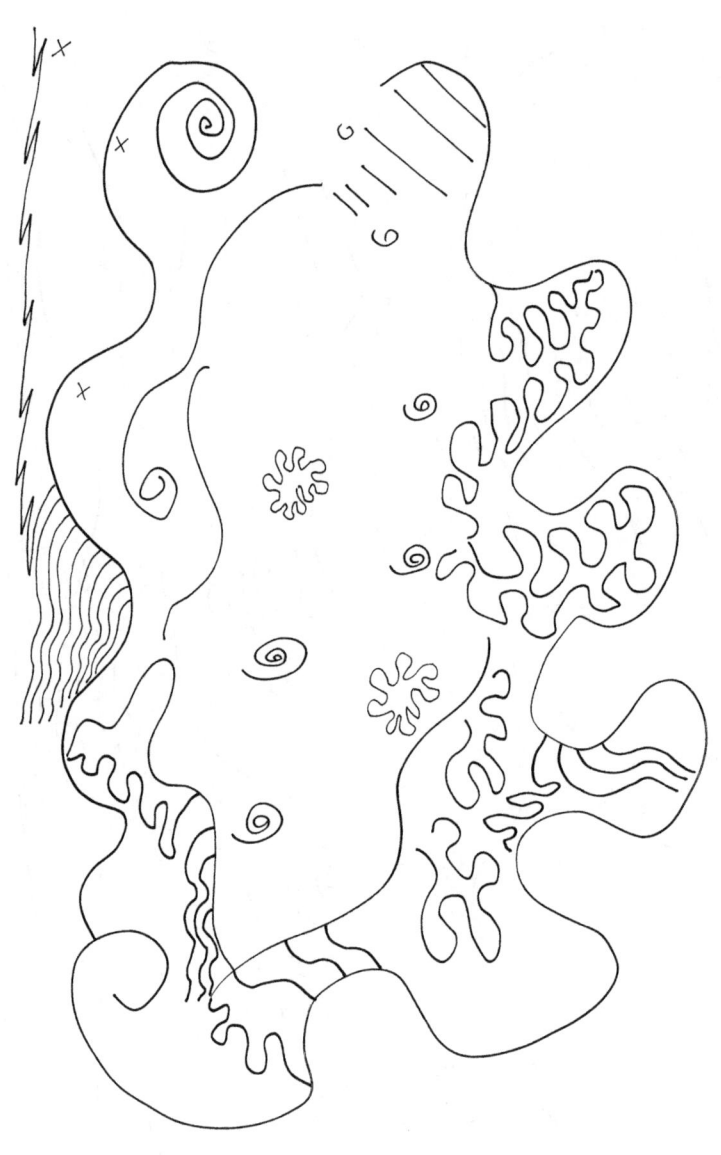

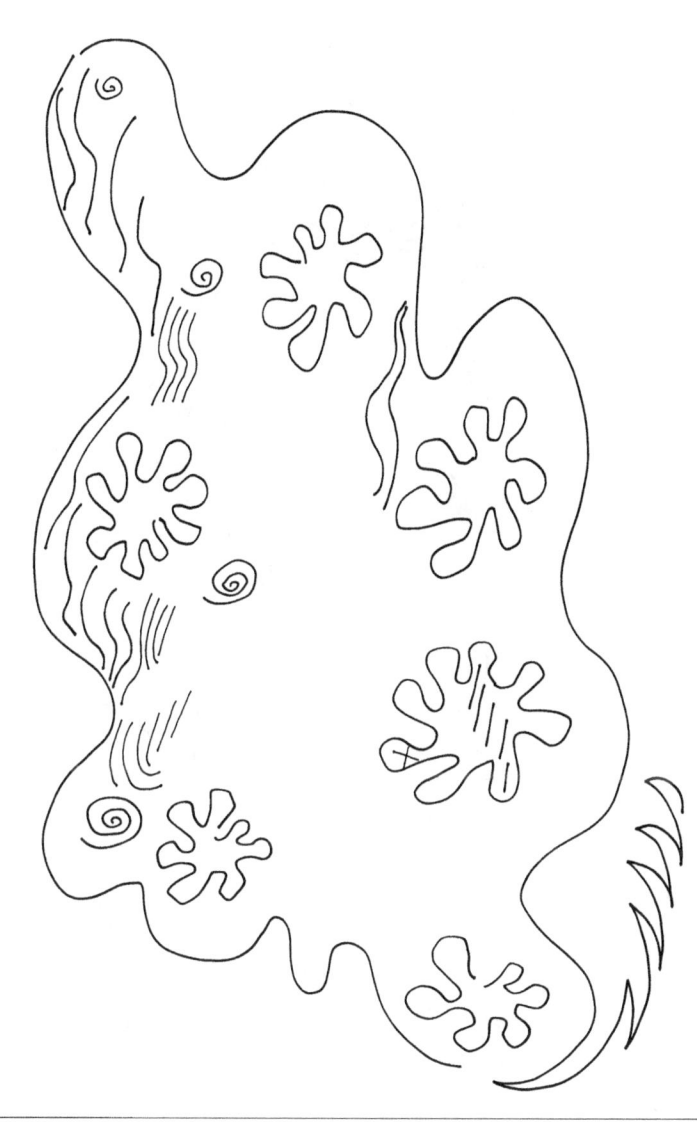

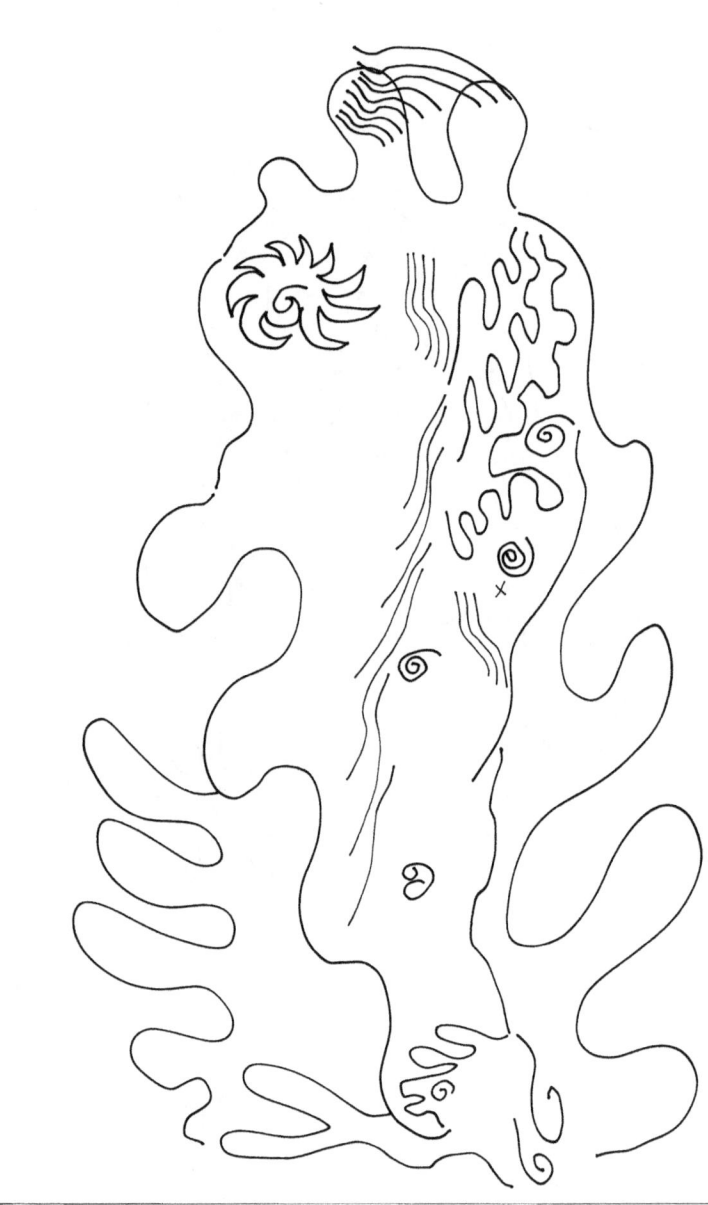

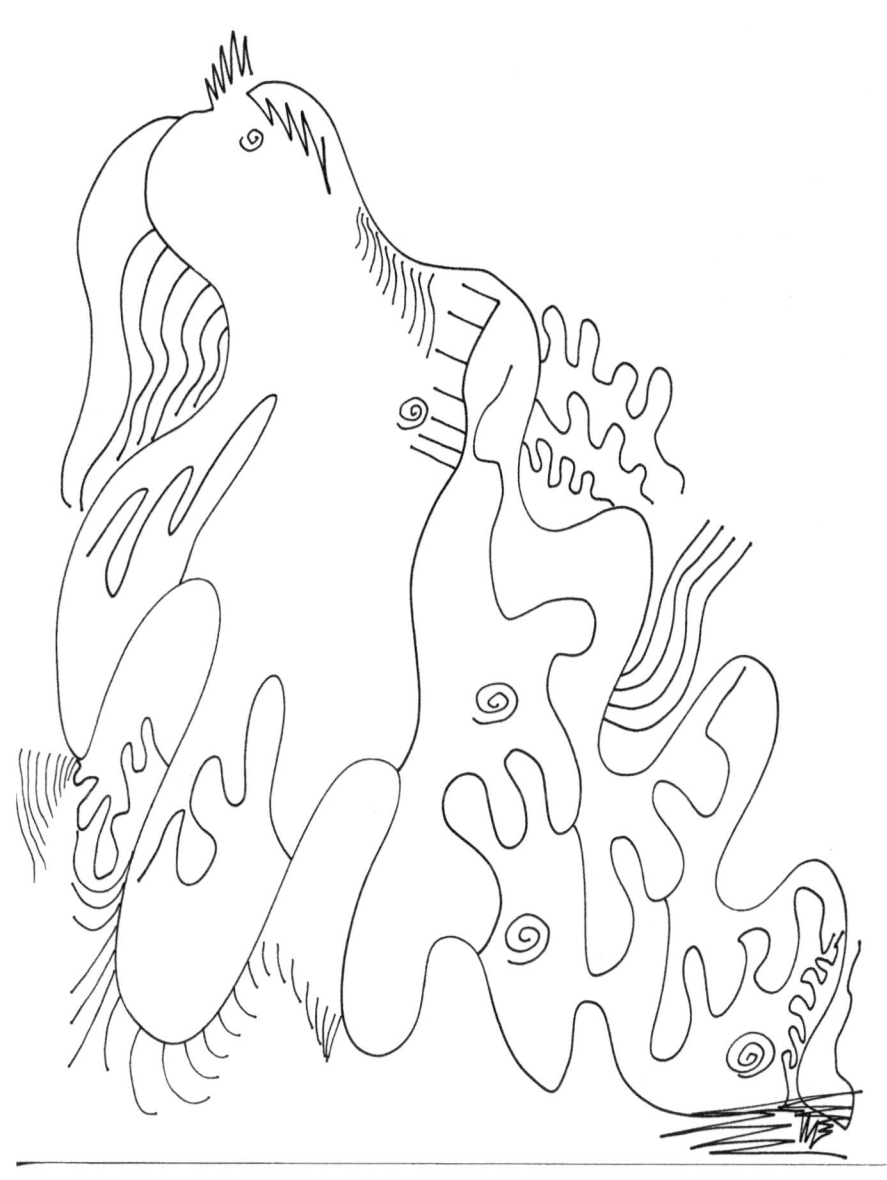

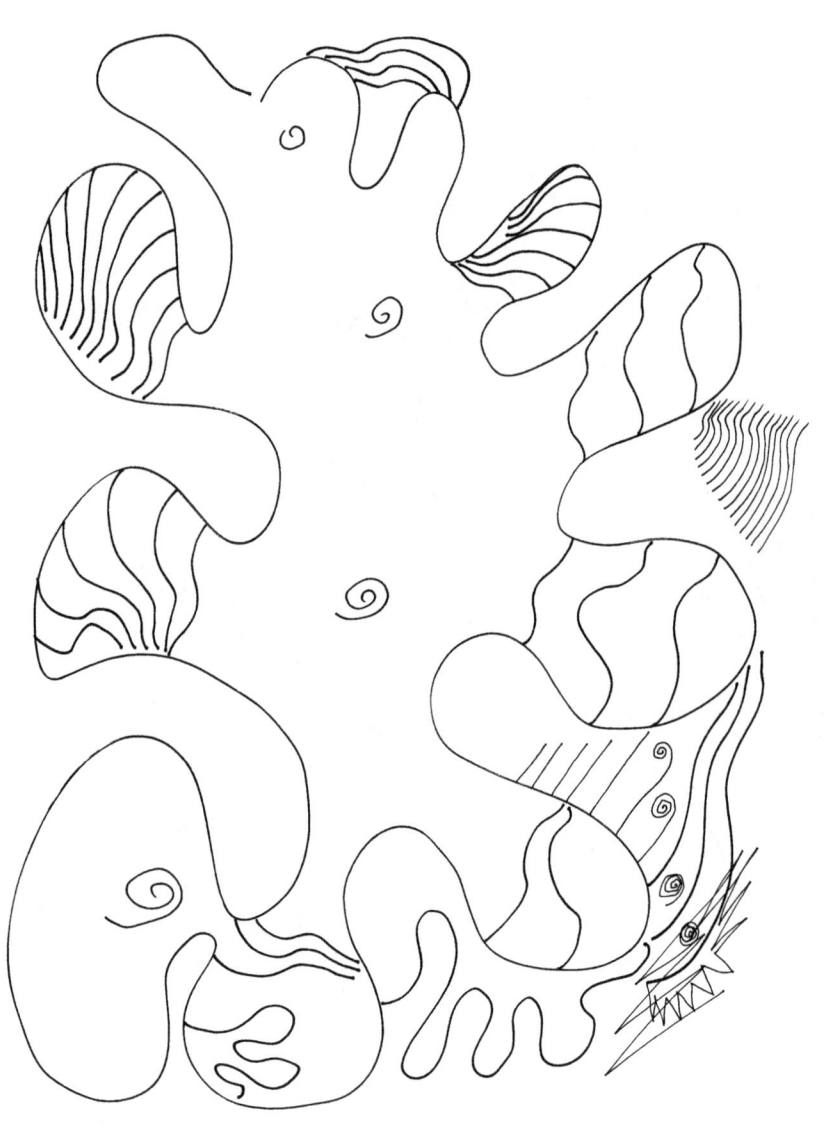

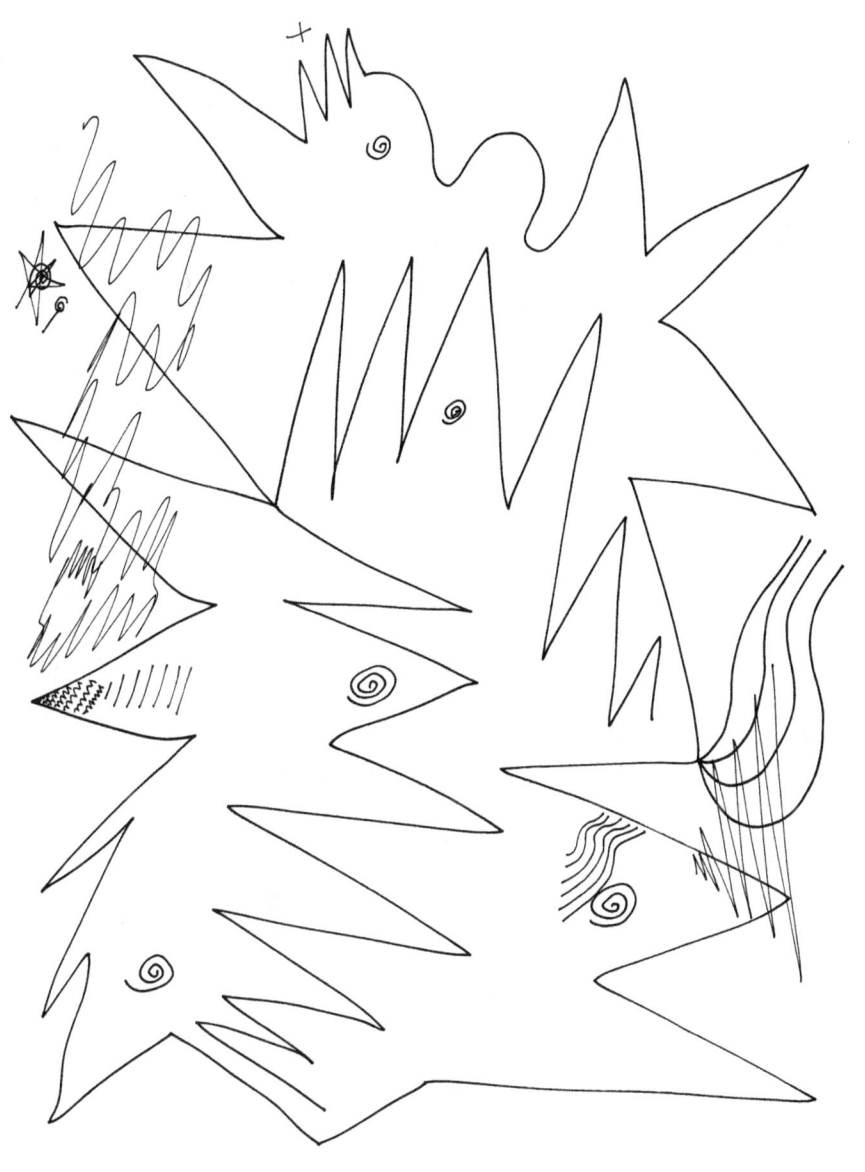

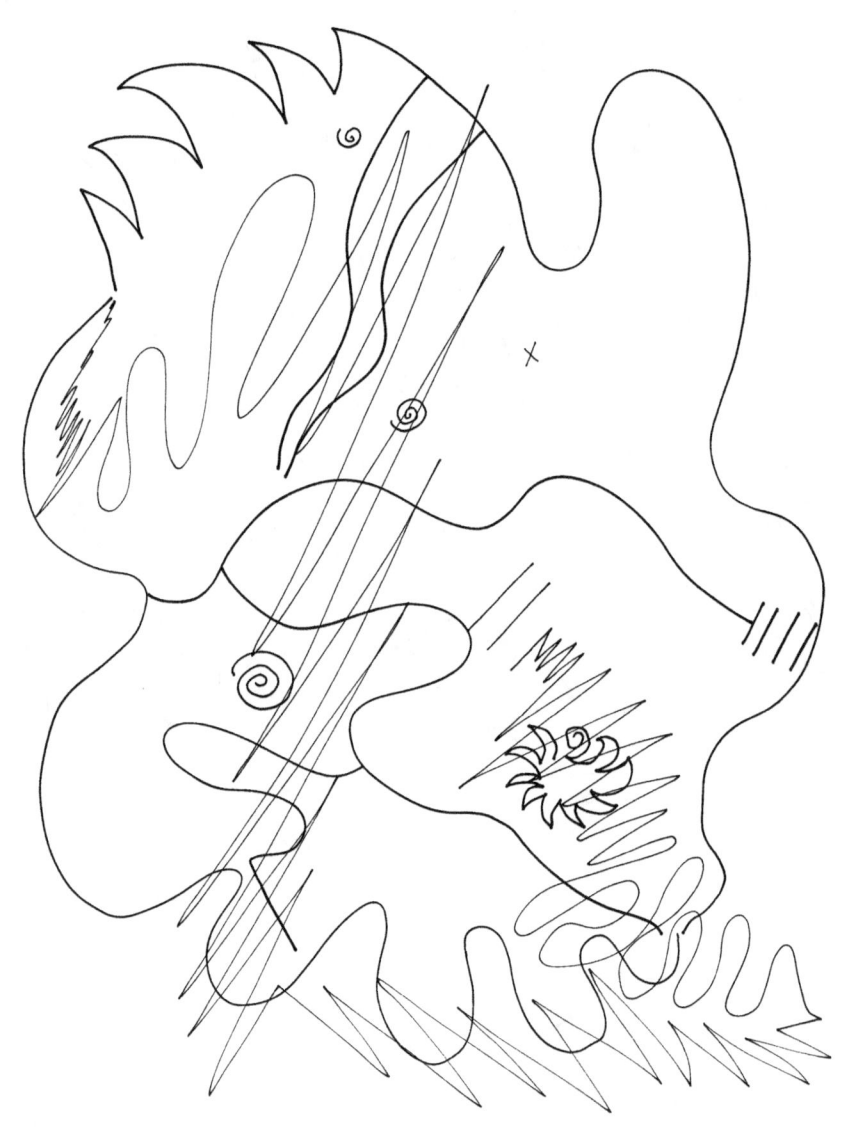

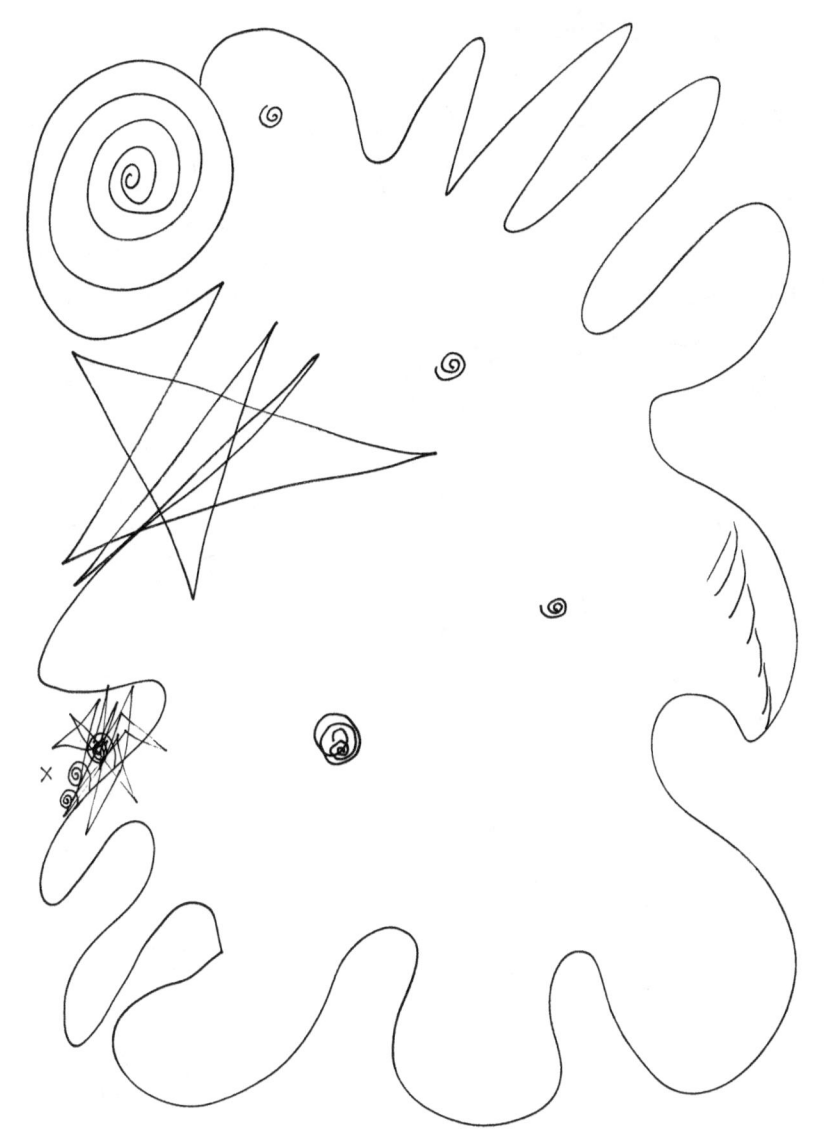

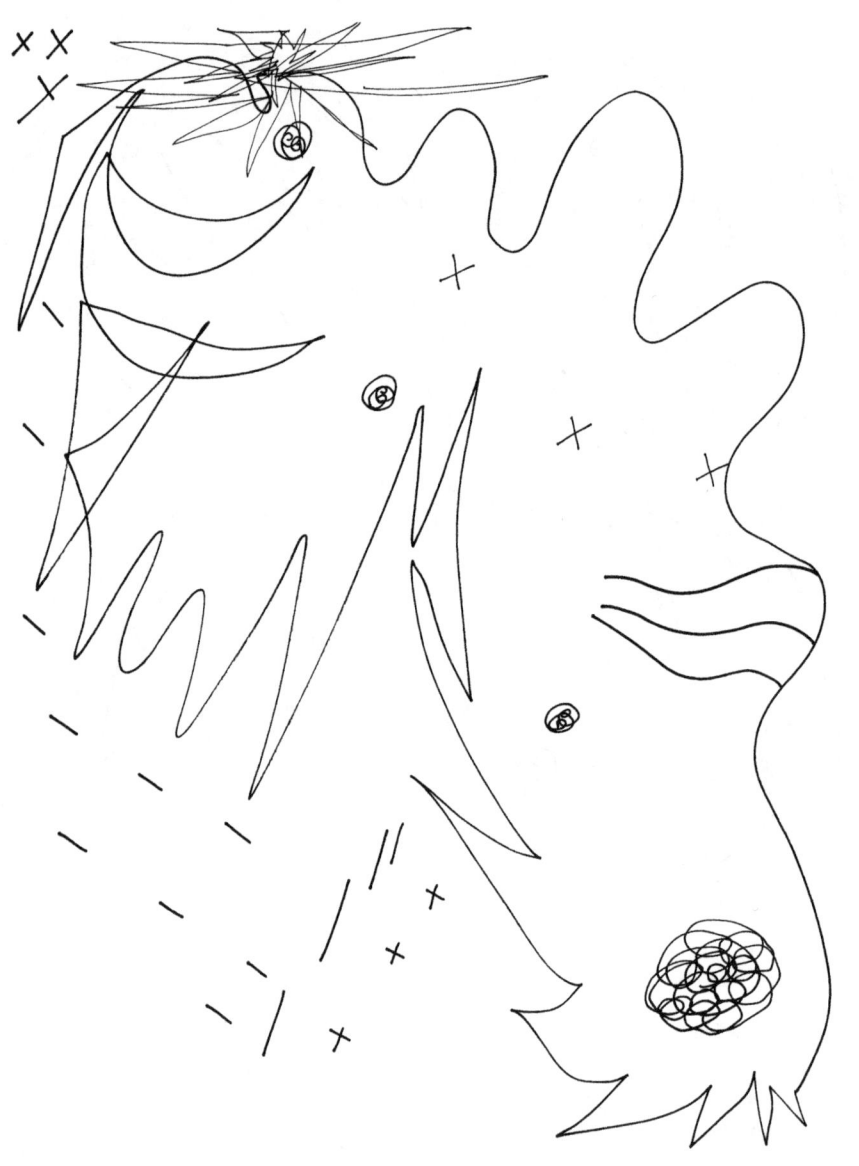

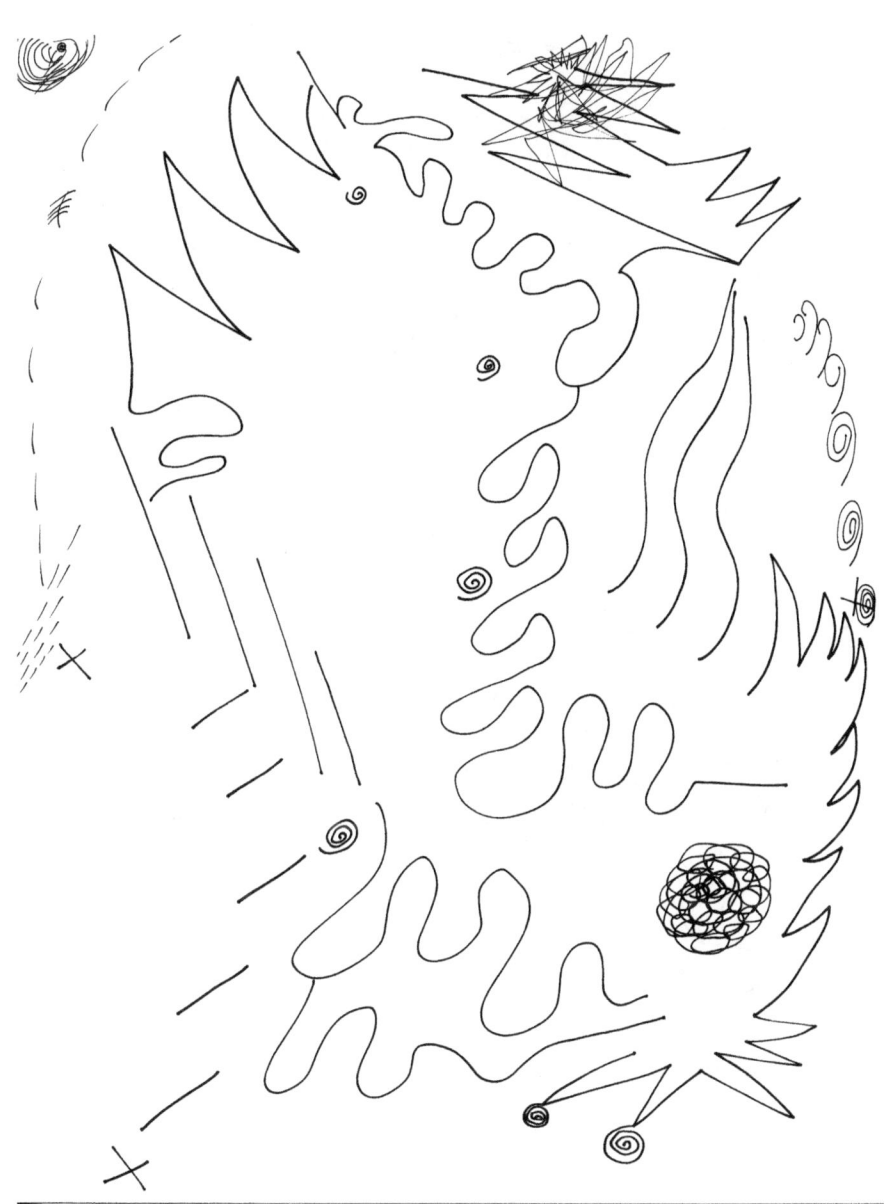

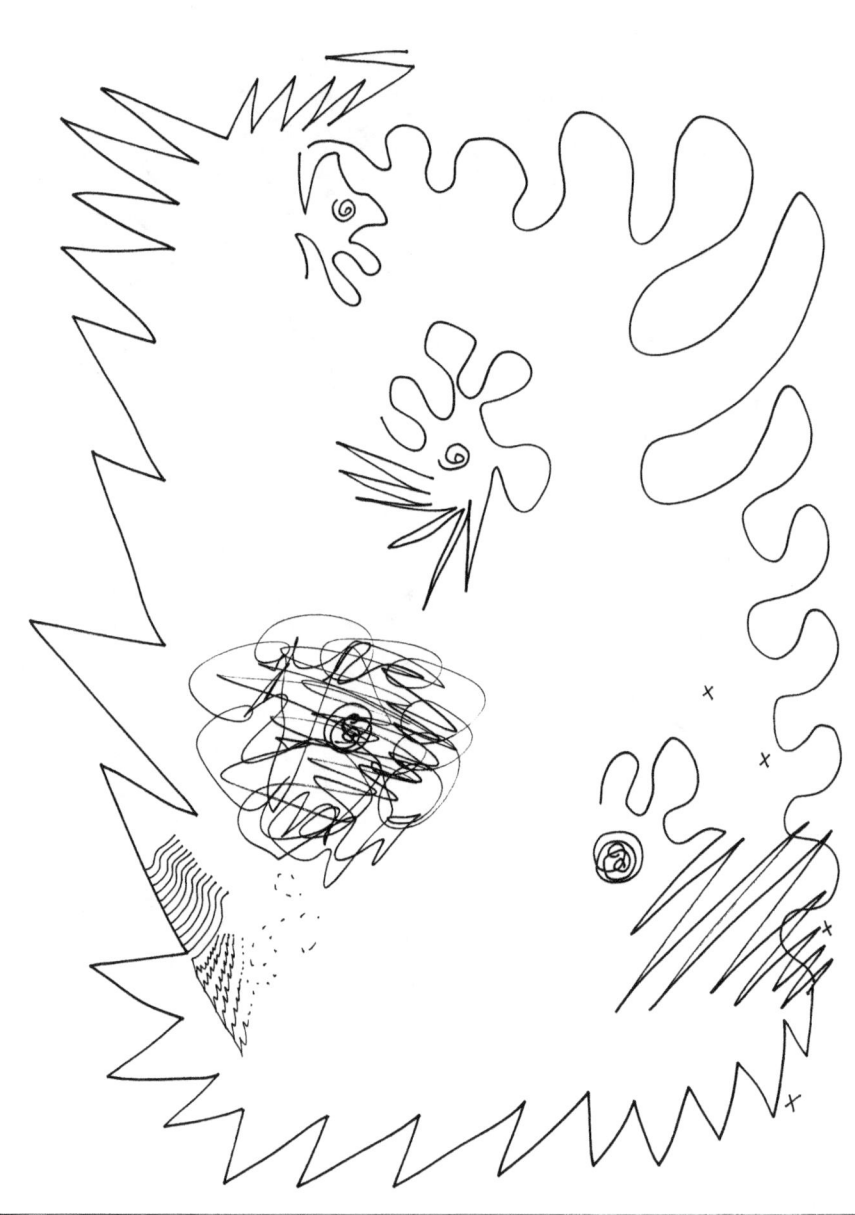

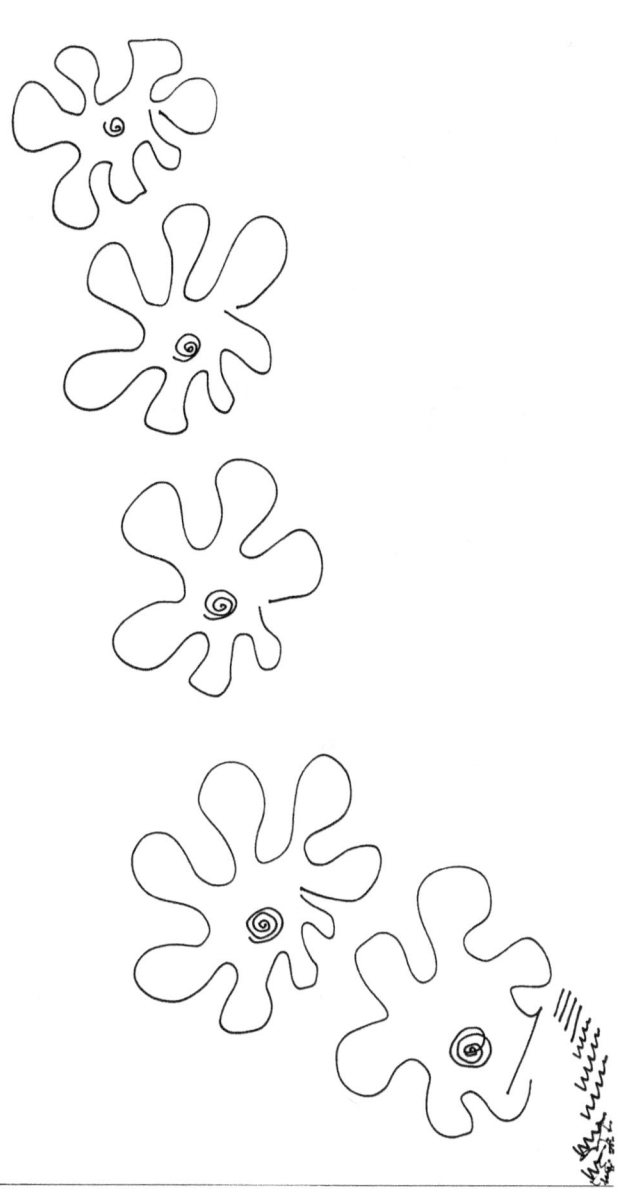

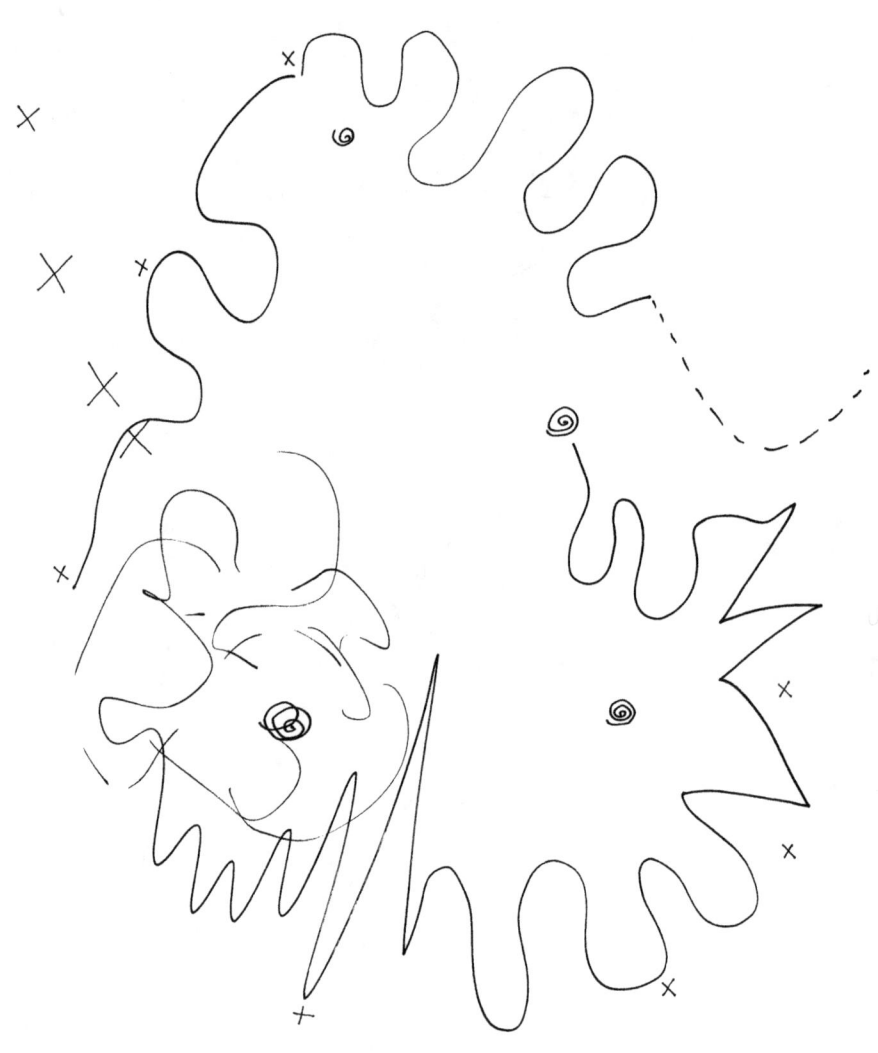

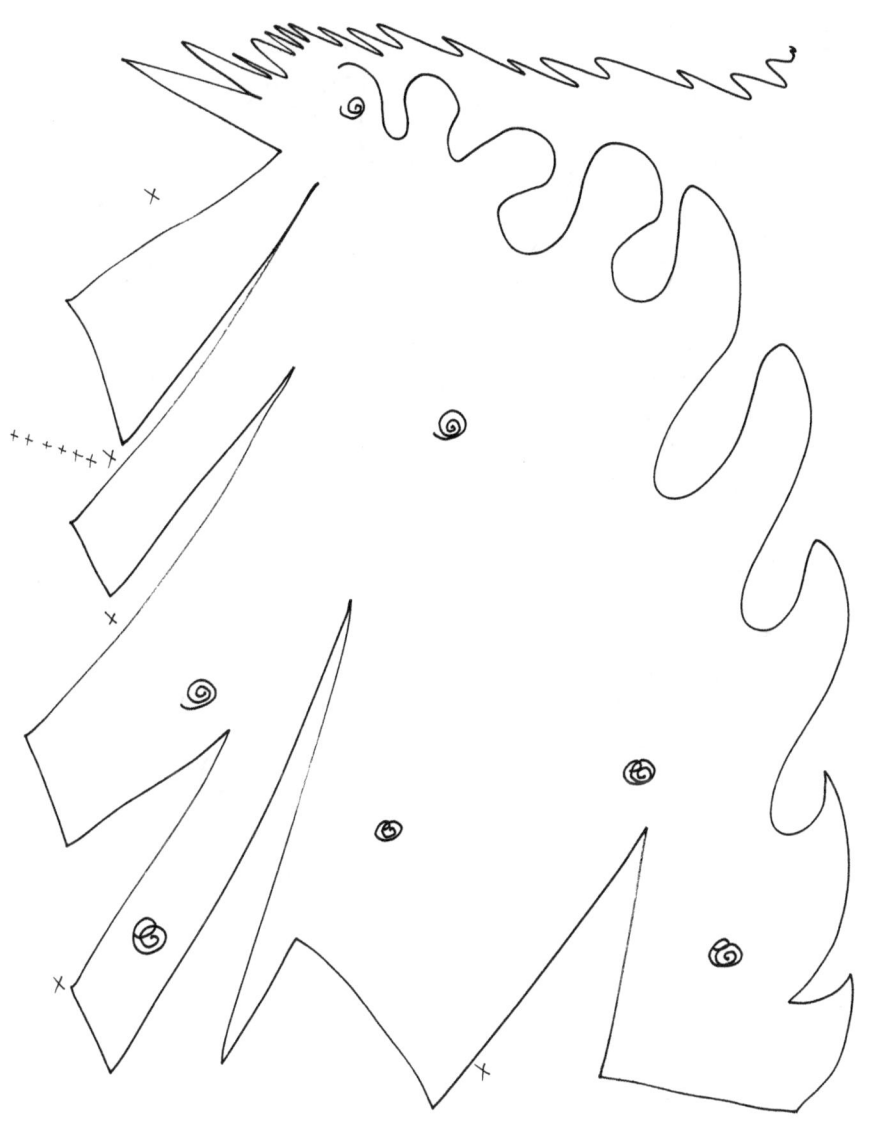

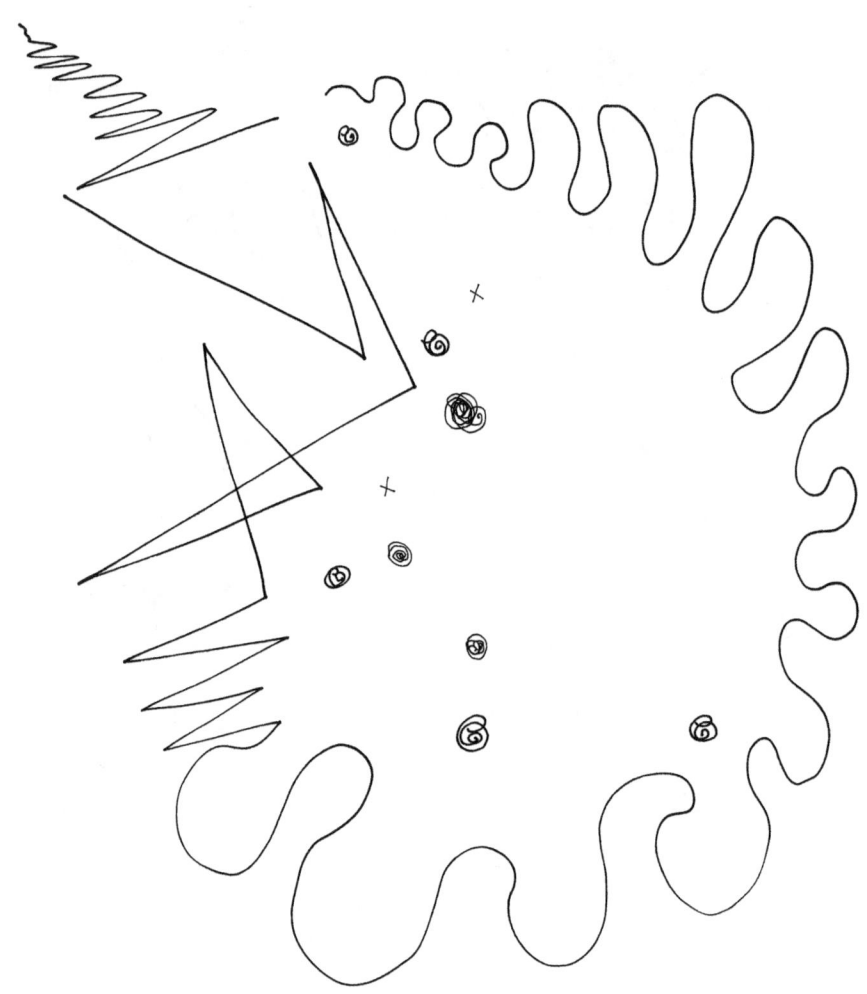

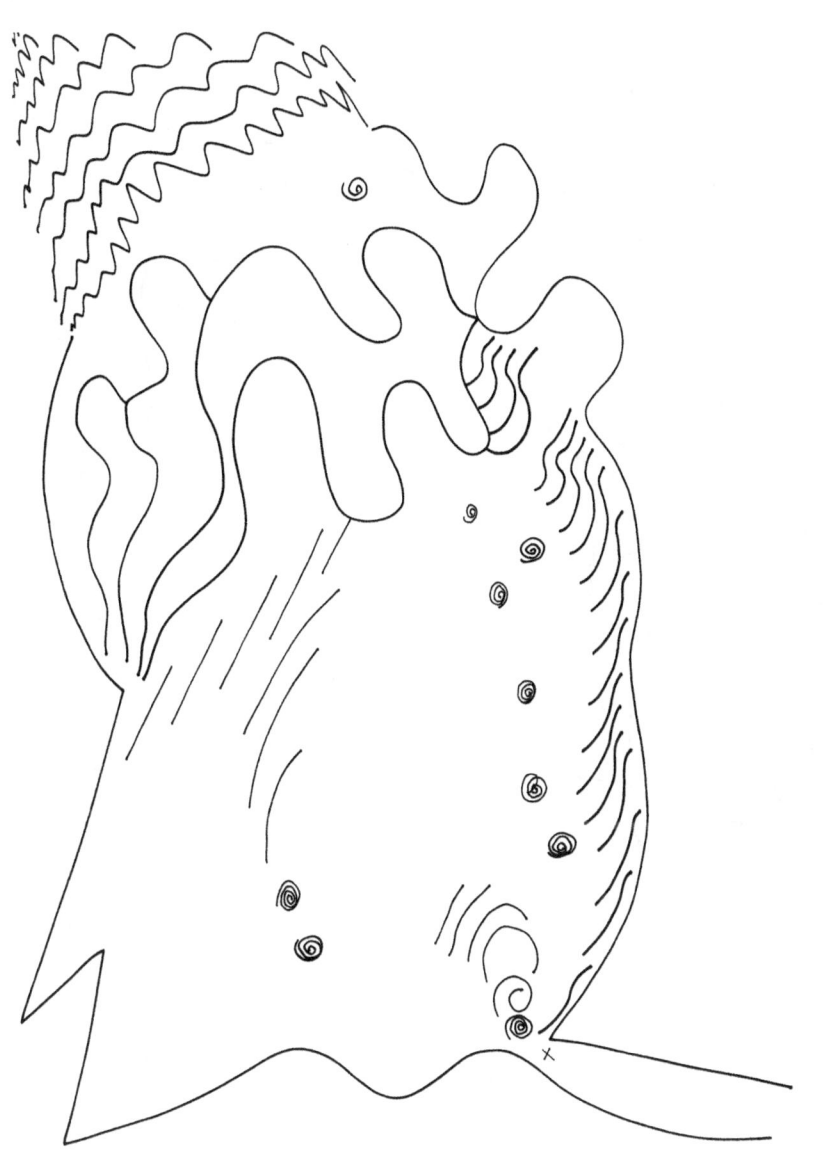

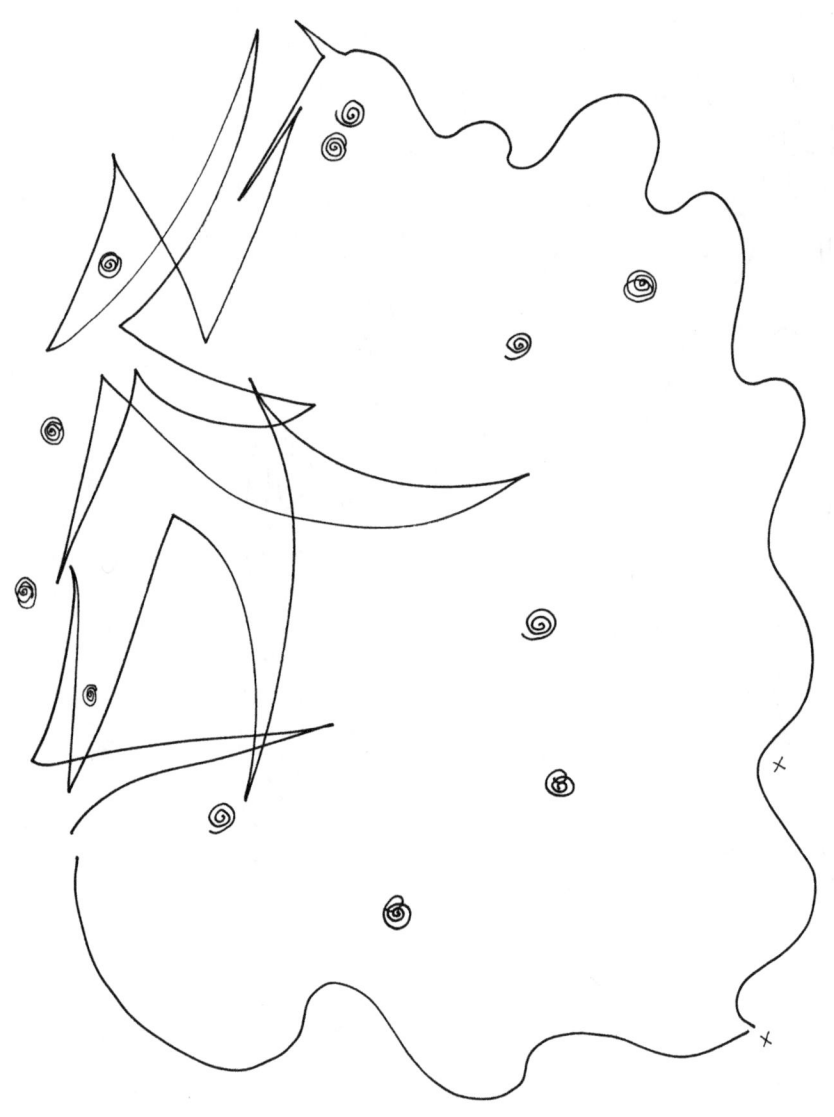

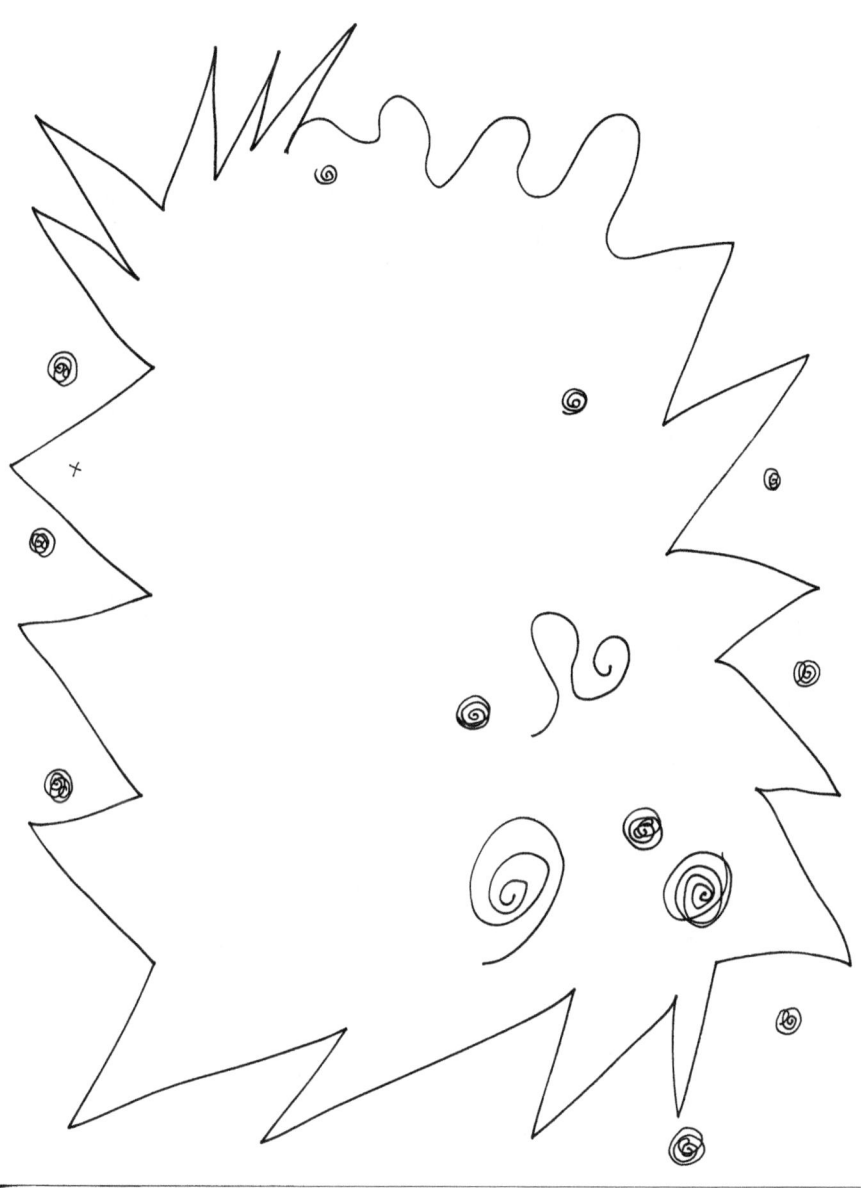

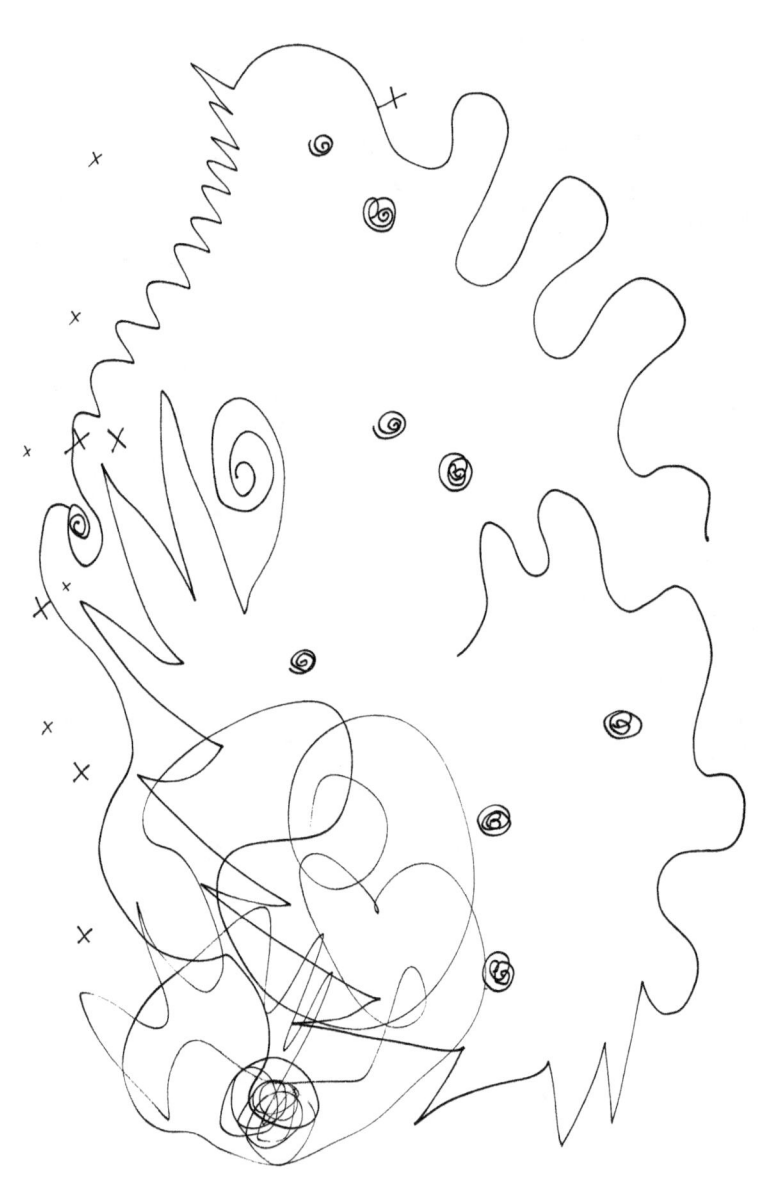

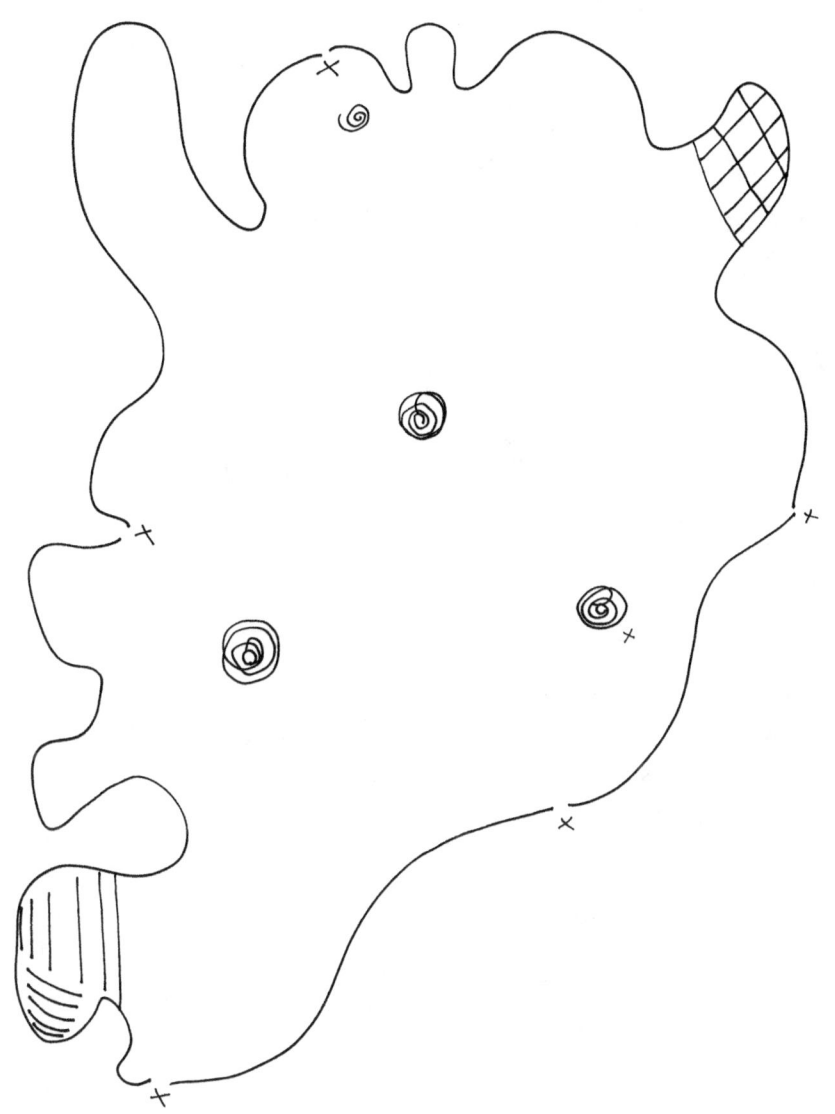

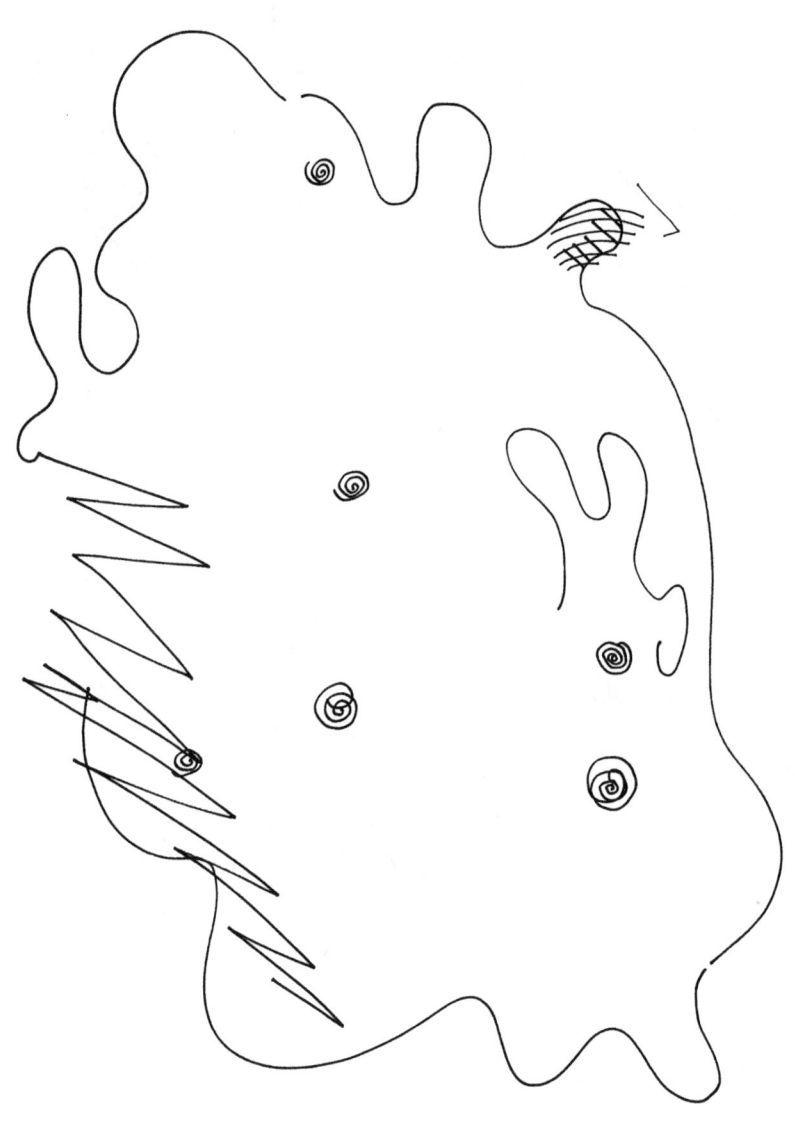

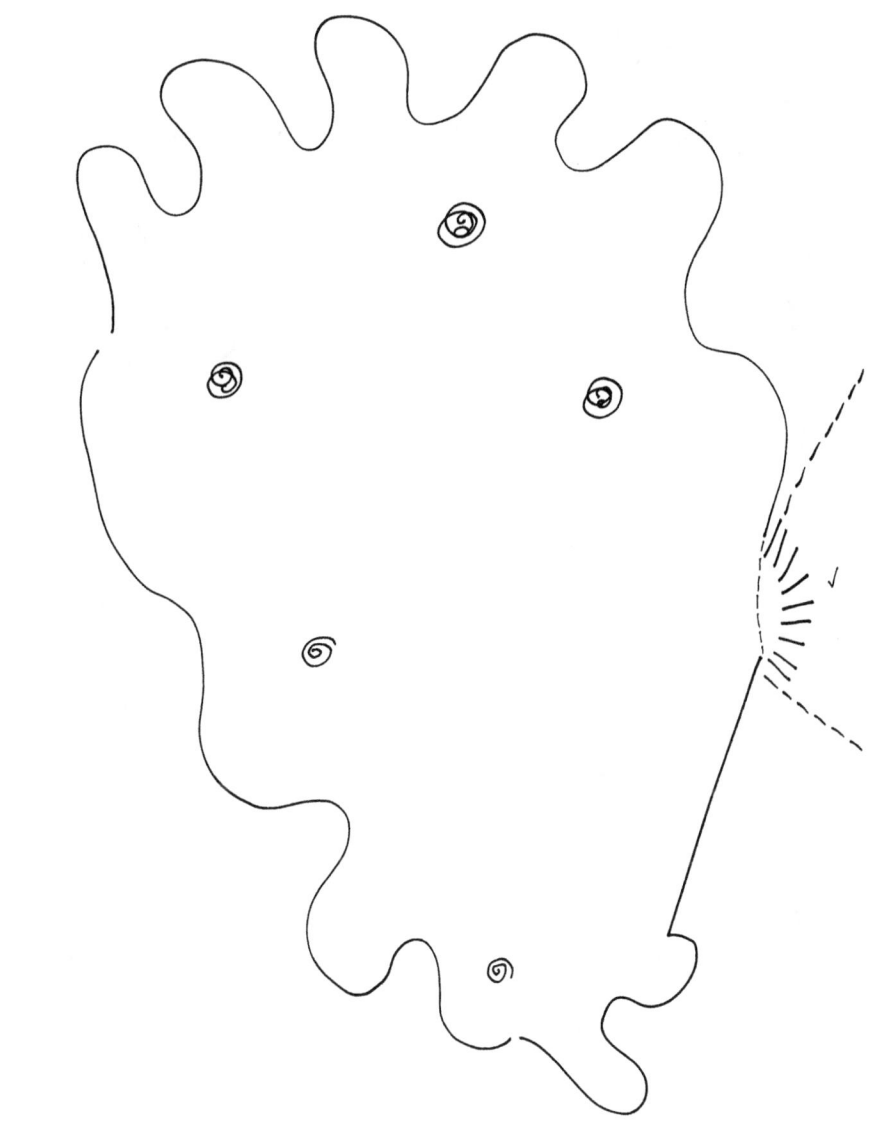

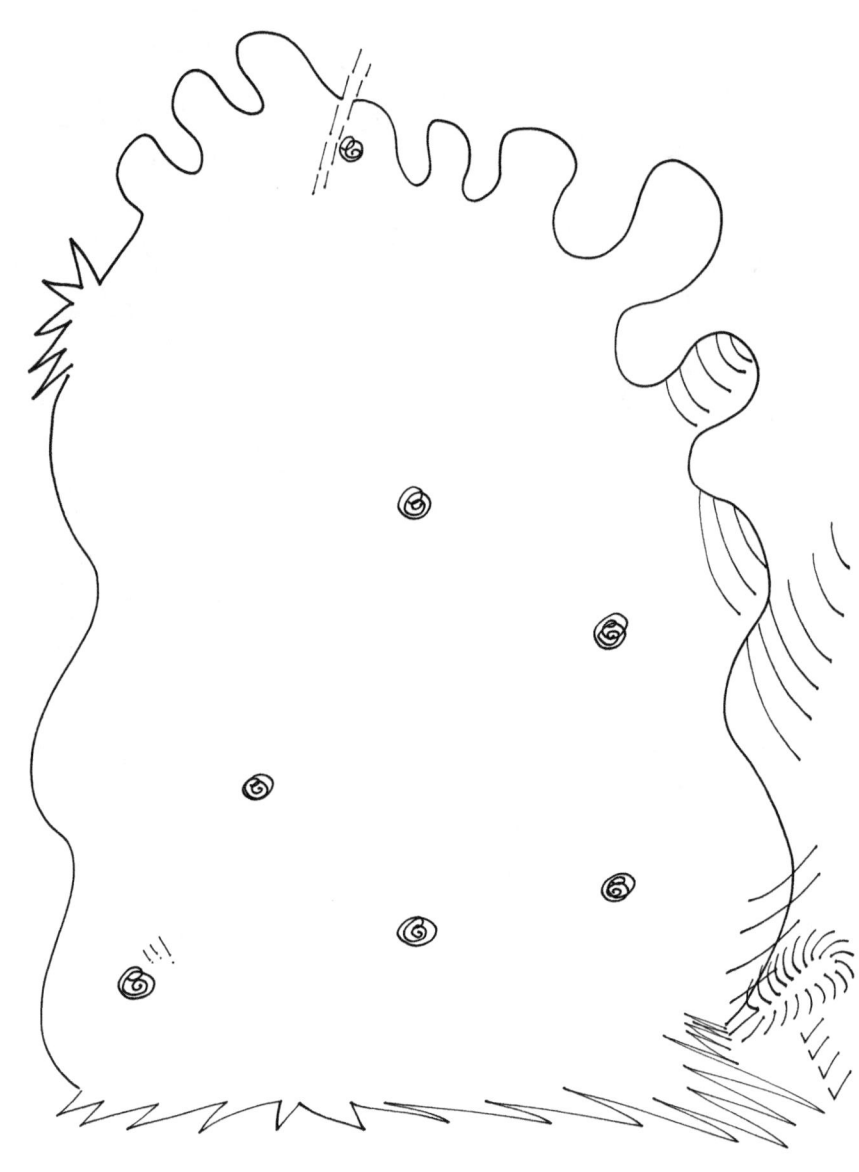

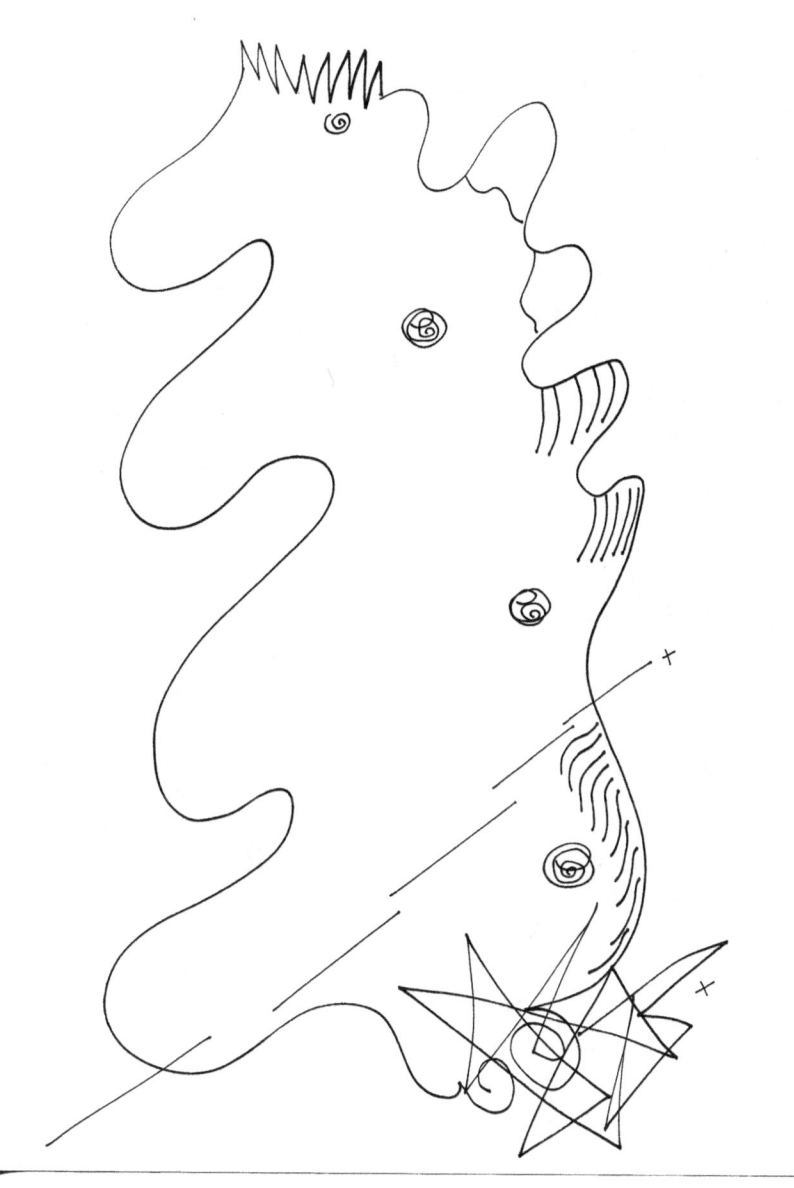

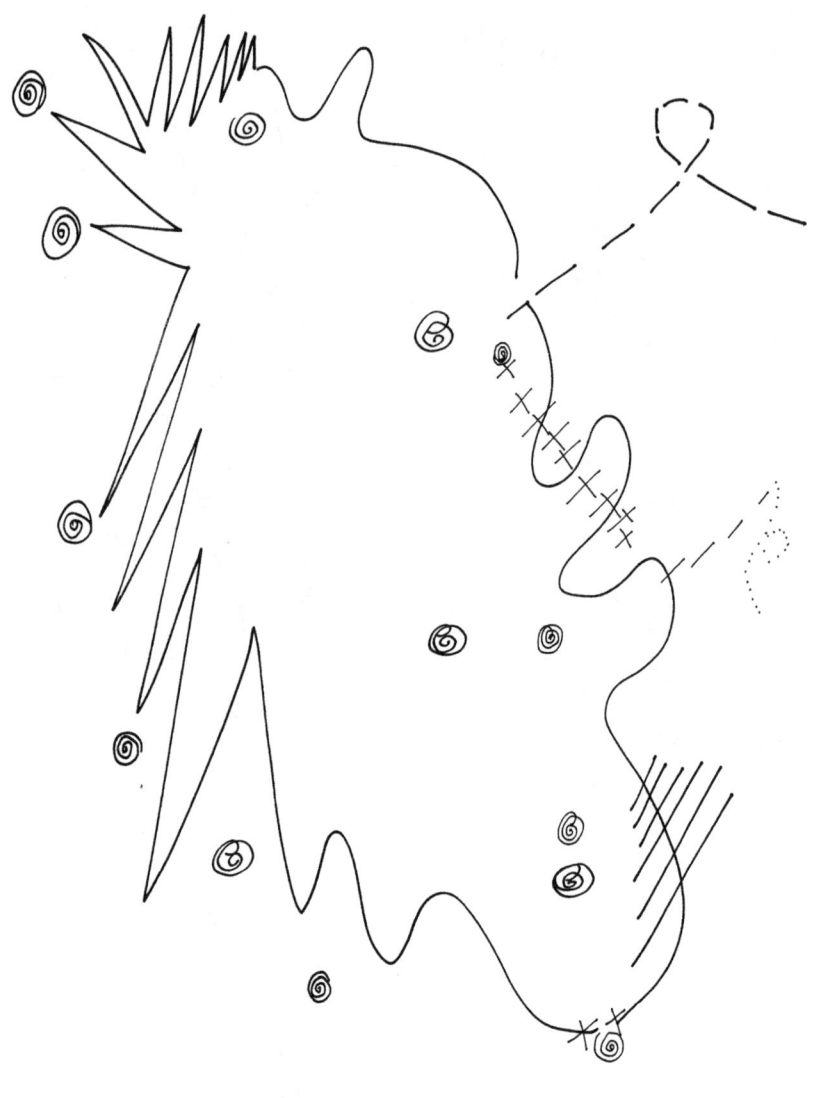

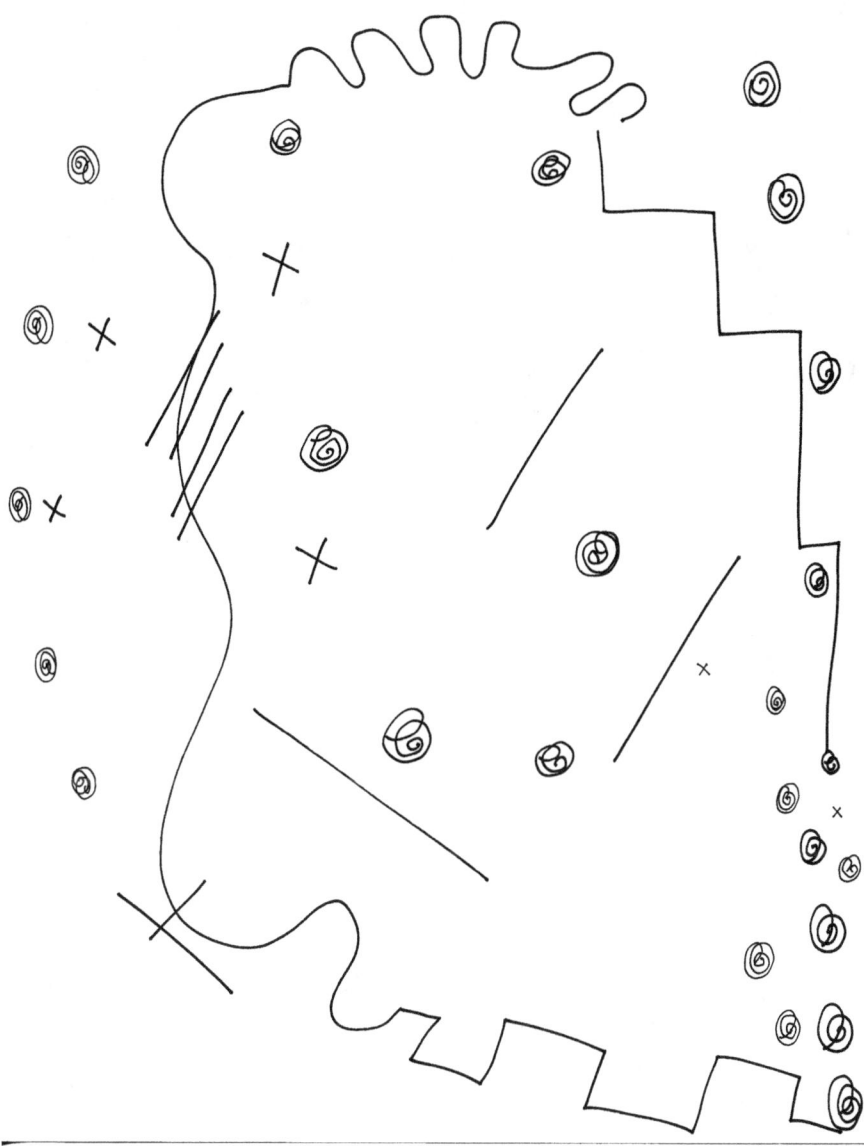

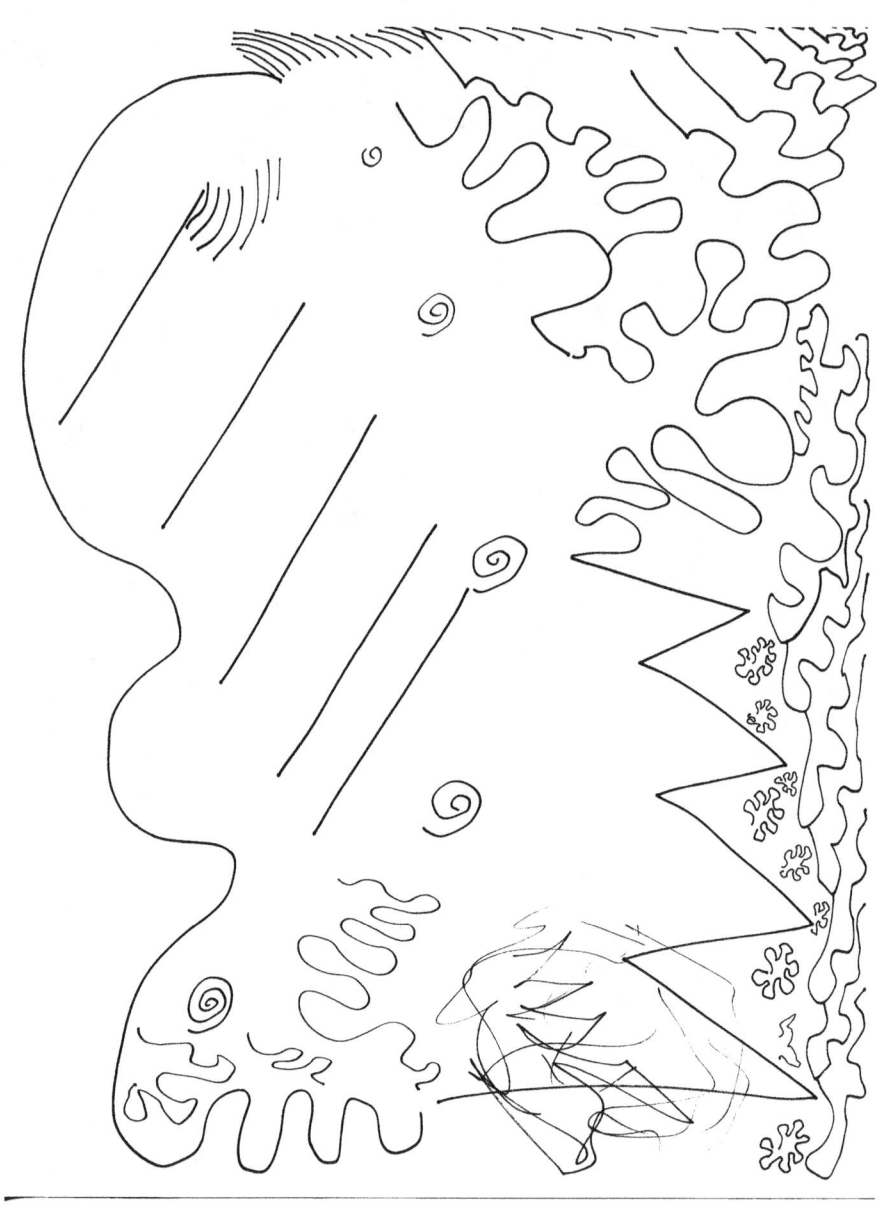

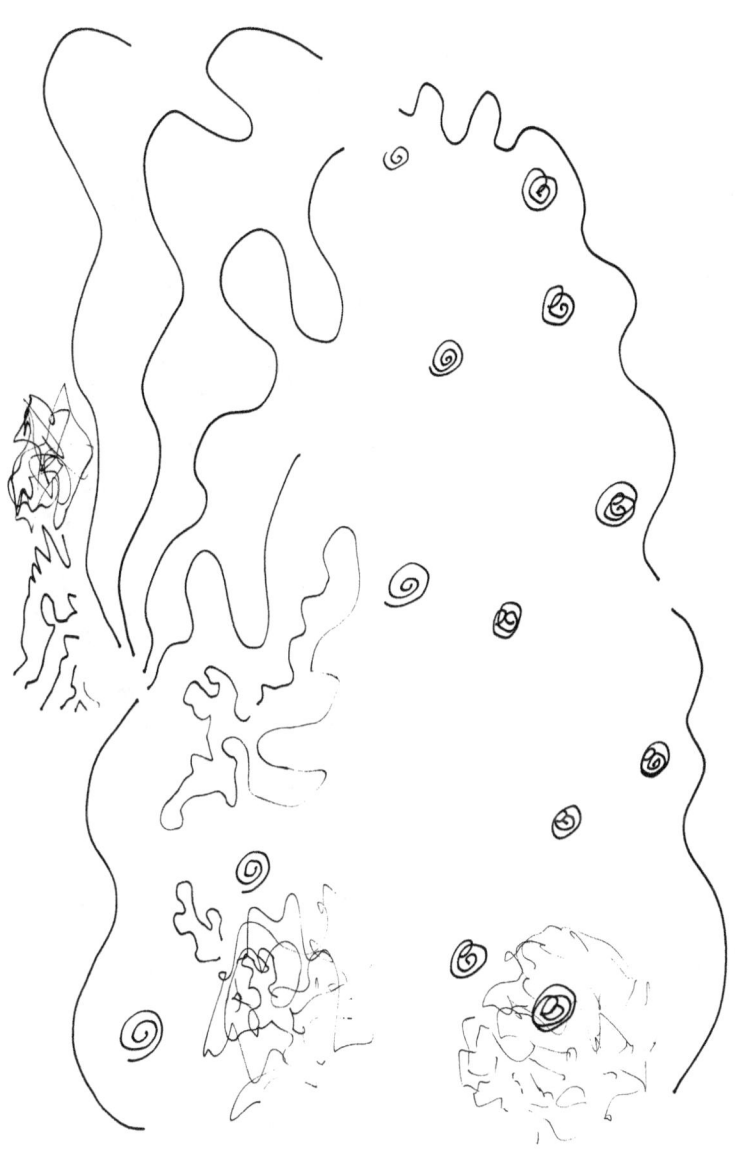

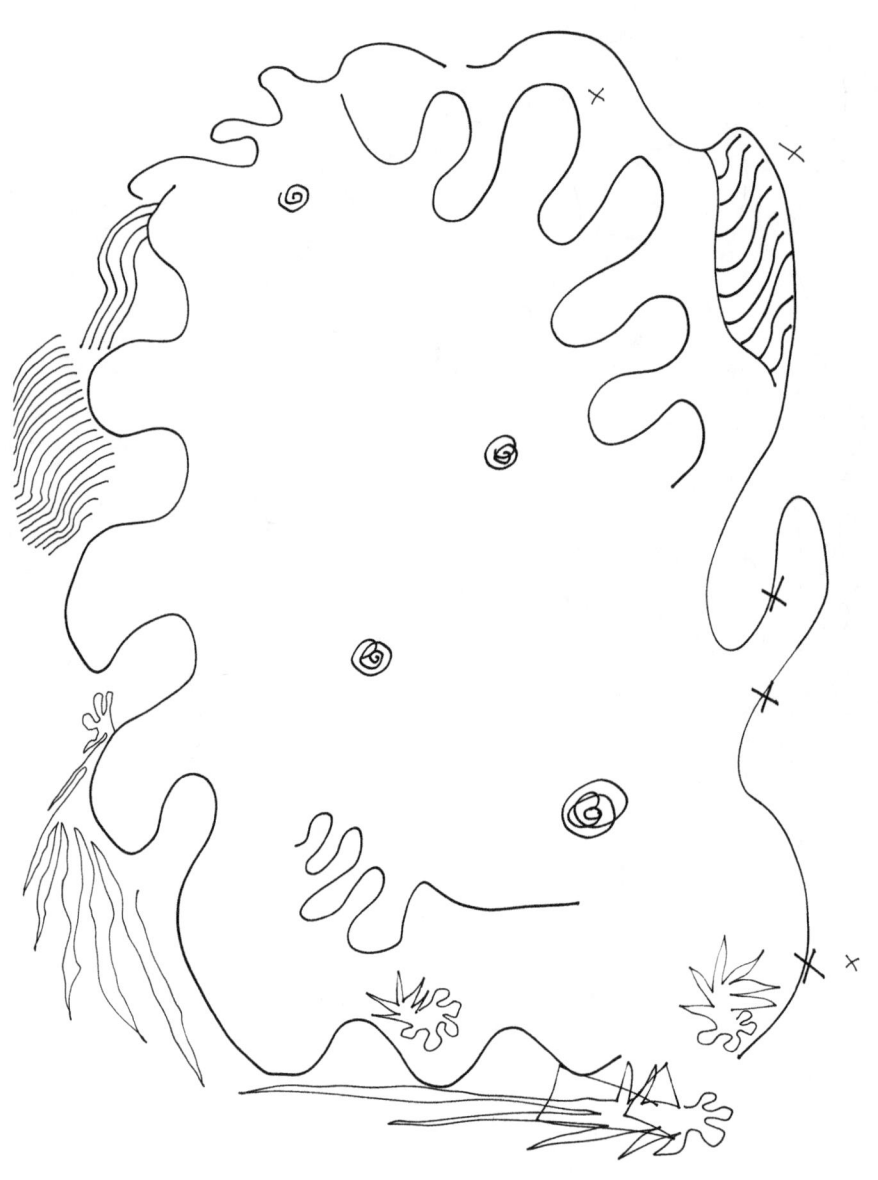

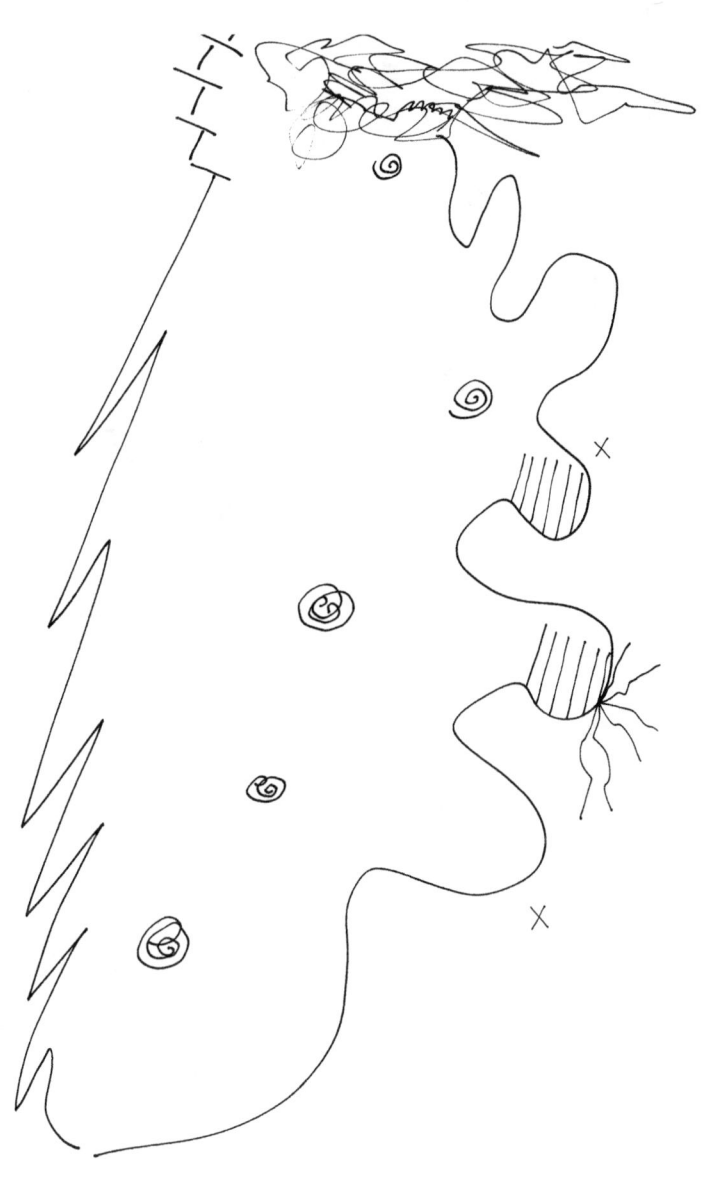

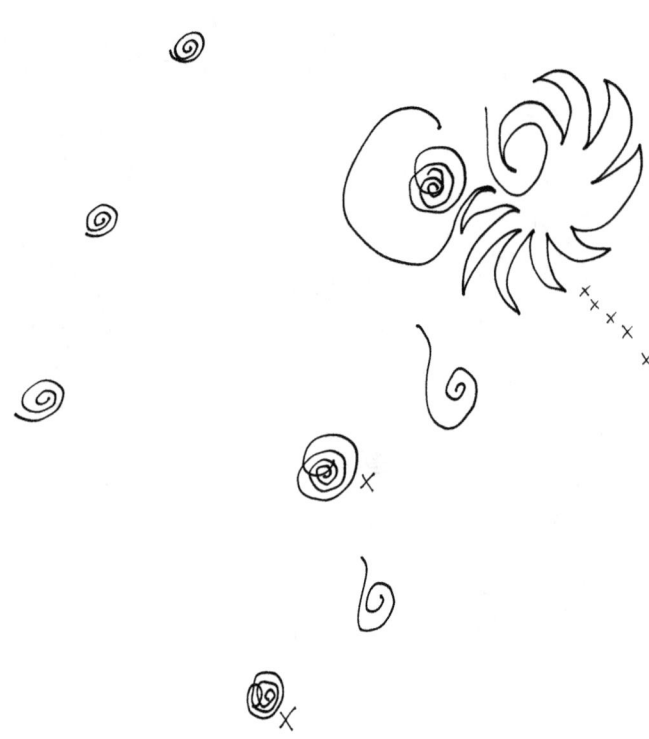

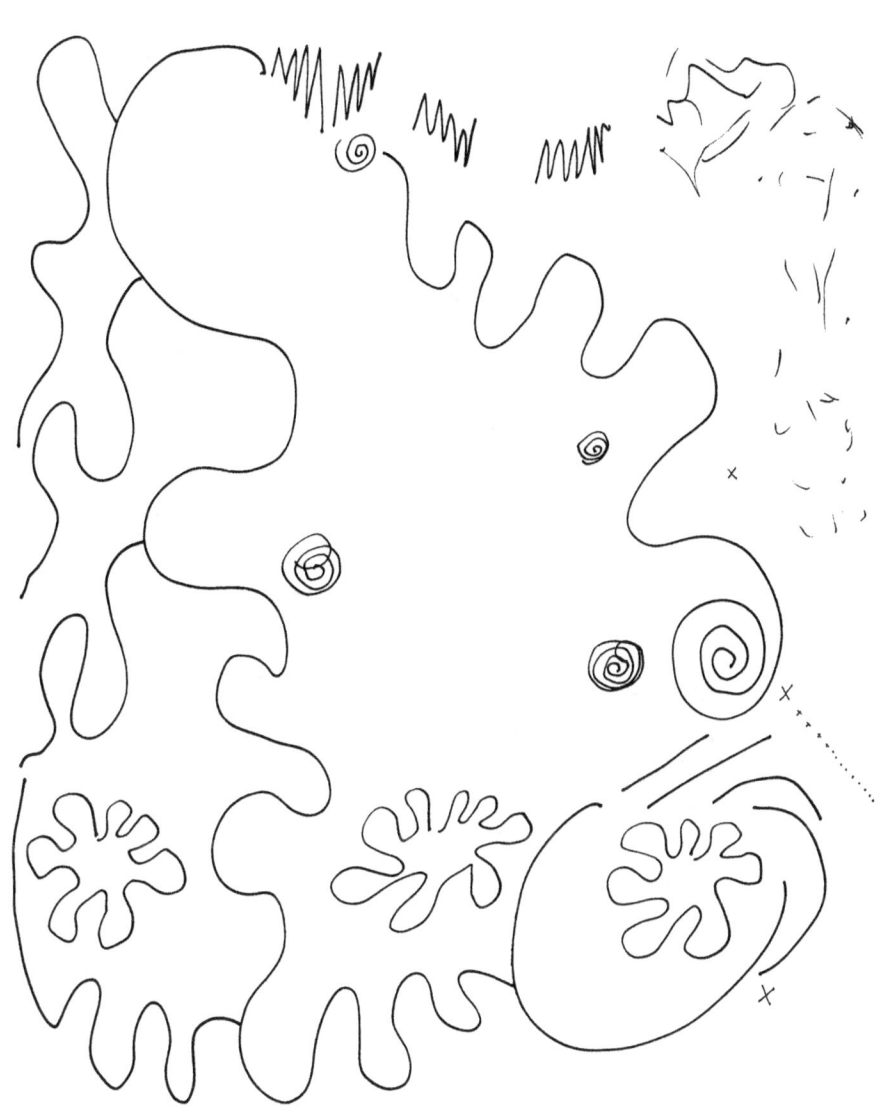

✓

 ✓

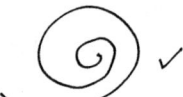 ✓

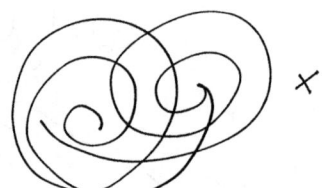 ✗

✓

 +

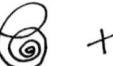 +

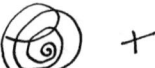 +

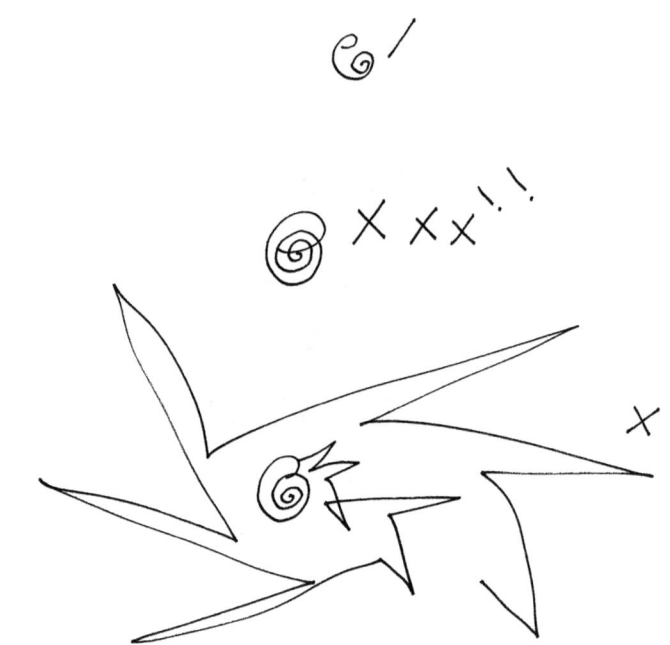

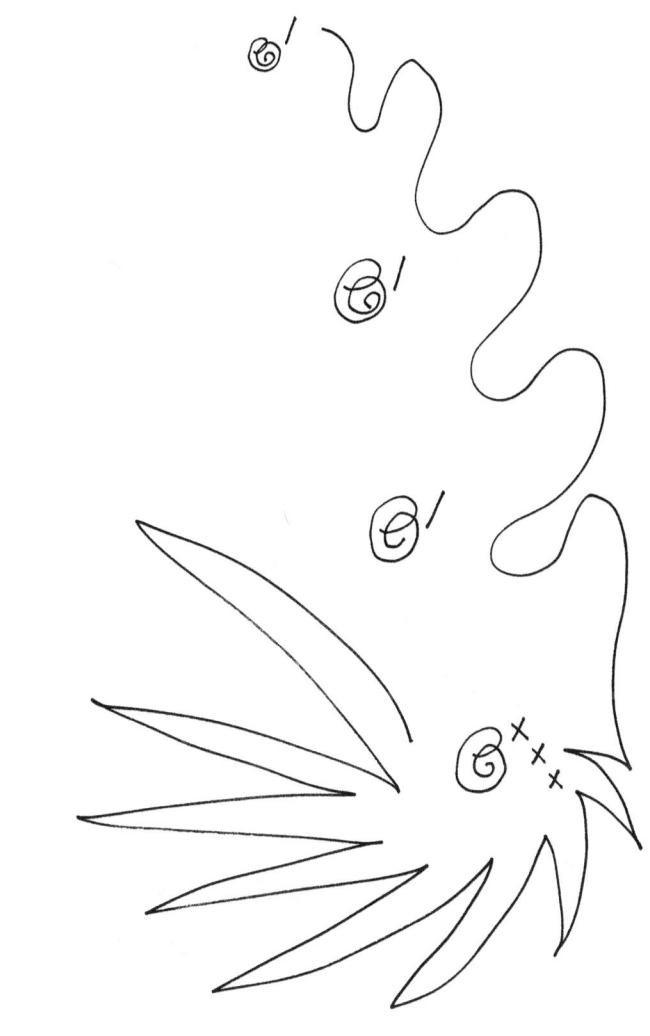

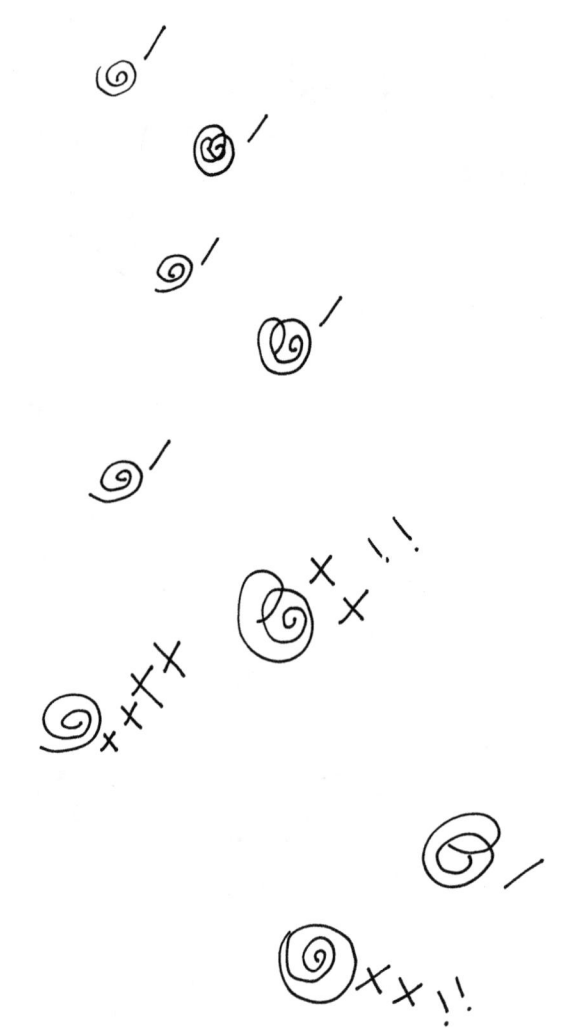

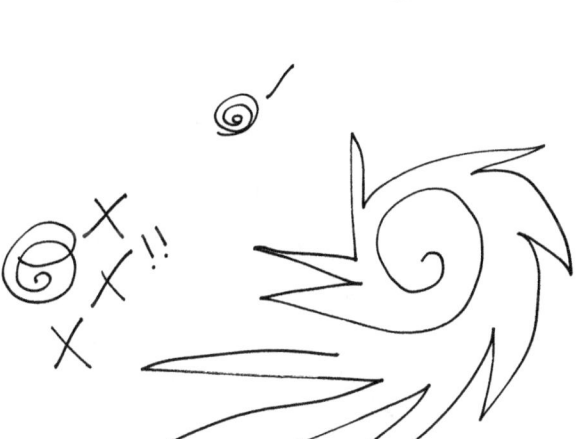

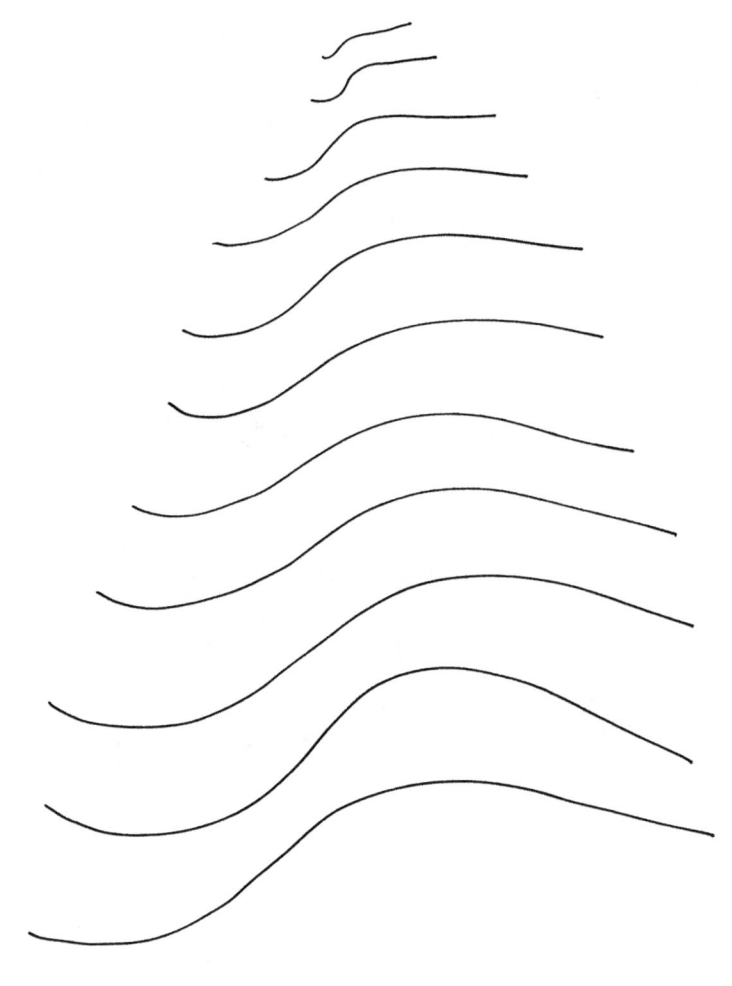

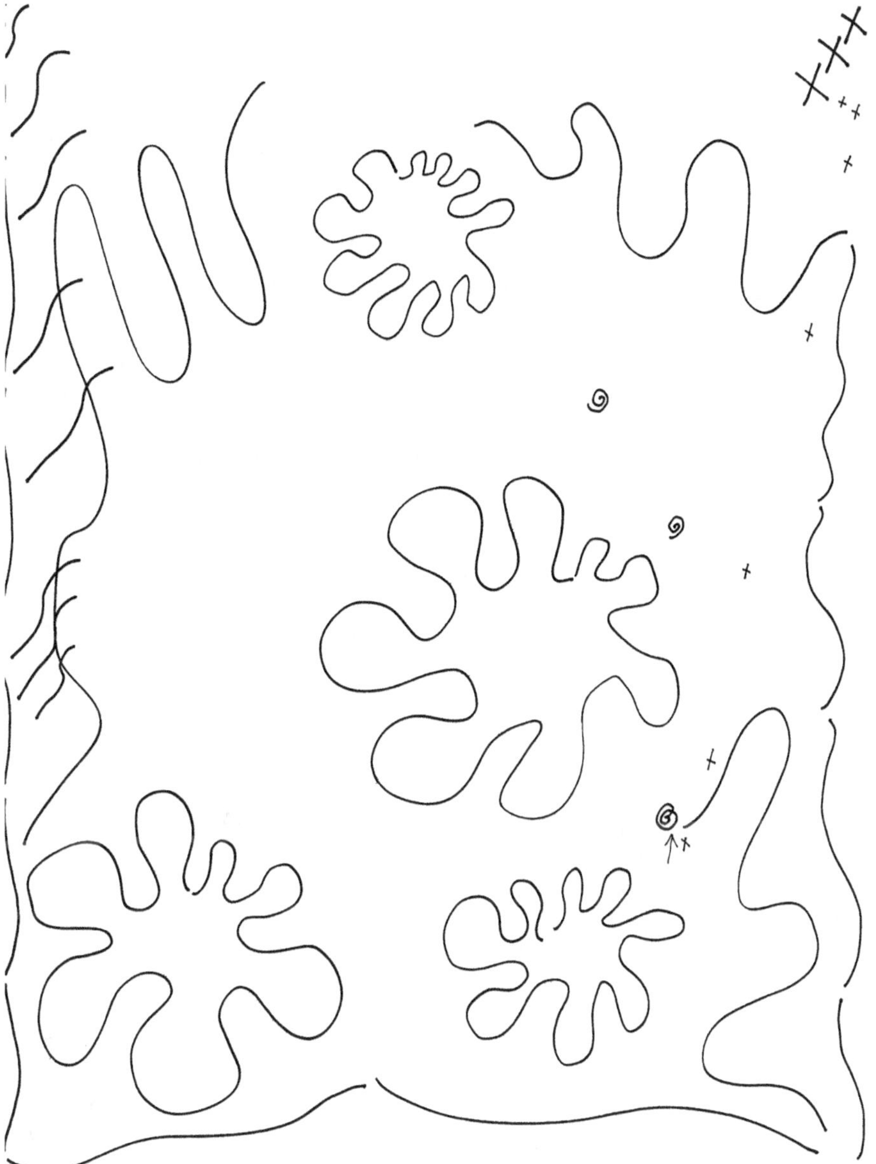

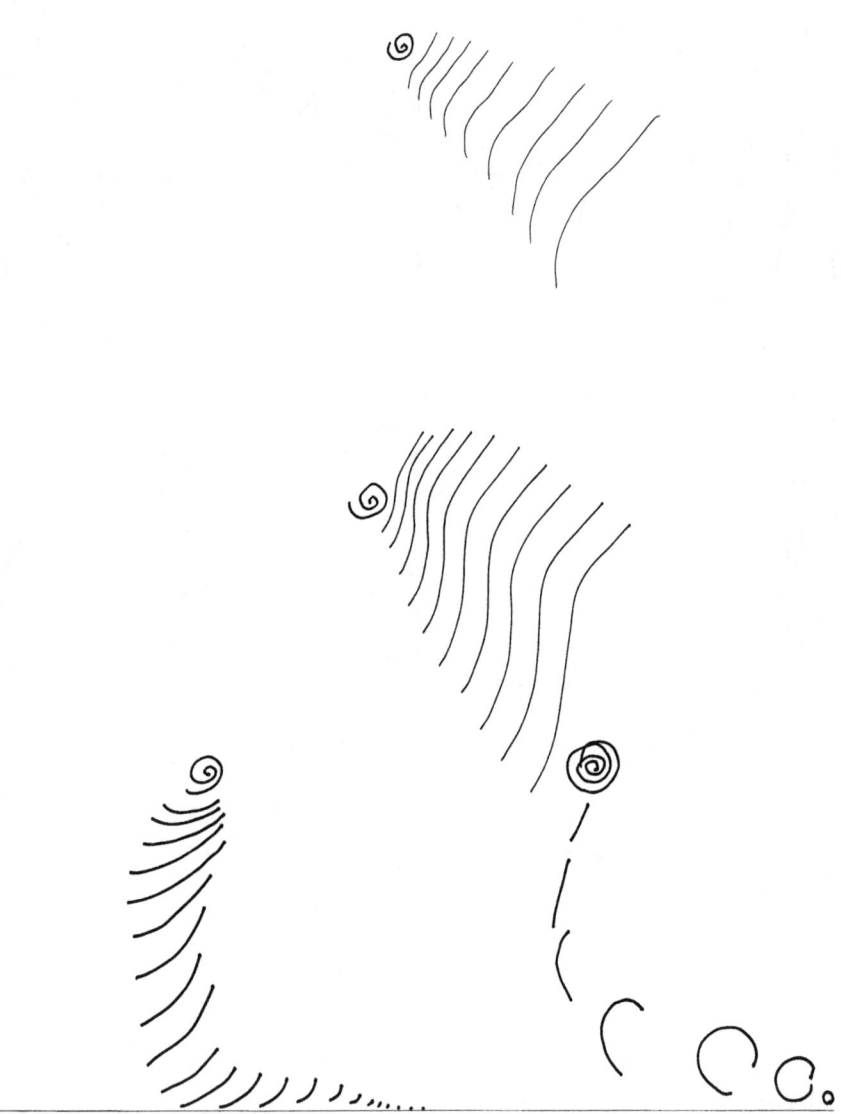

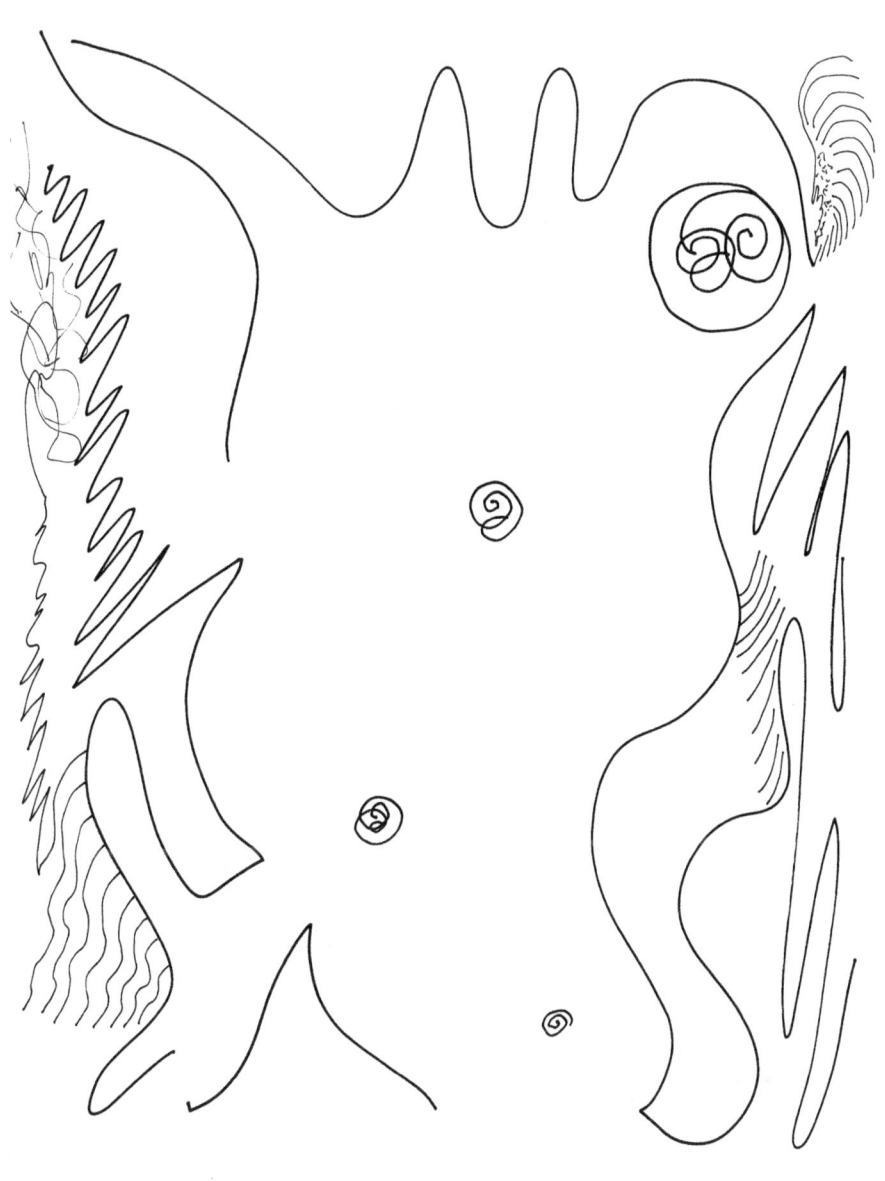

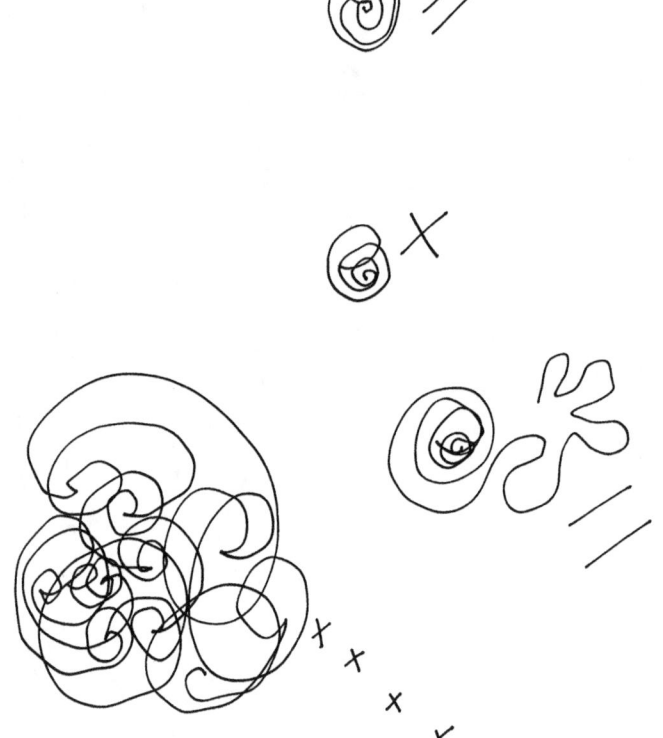

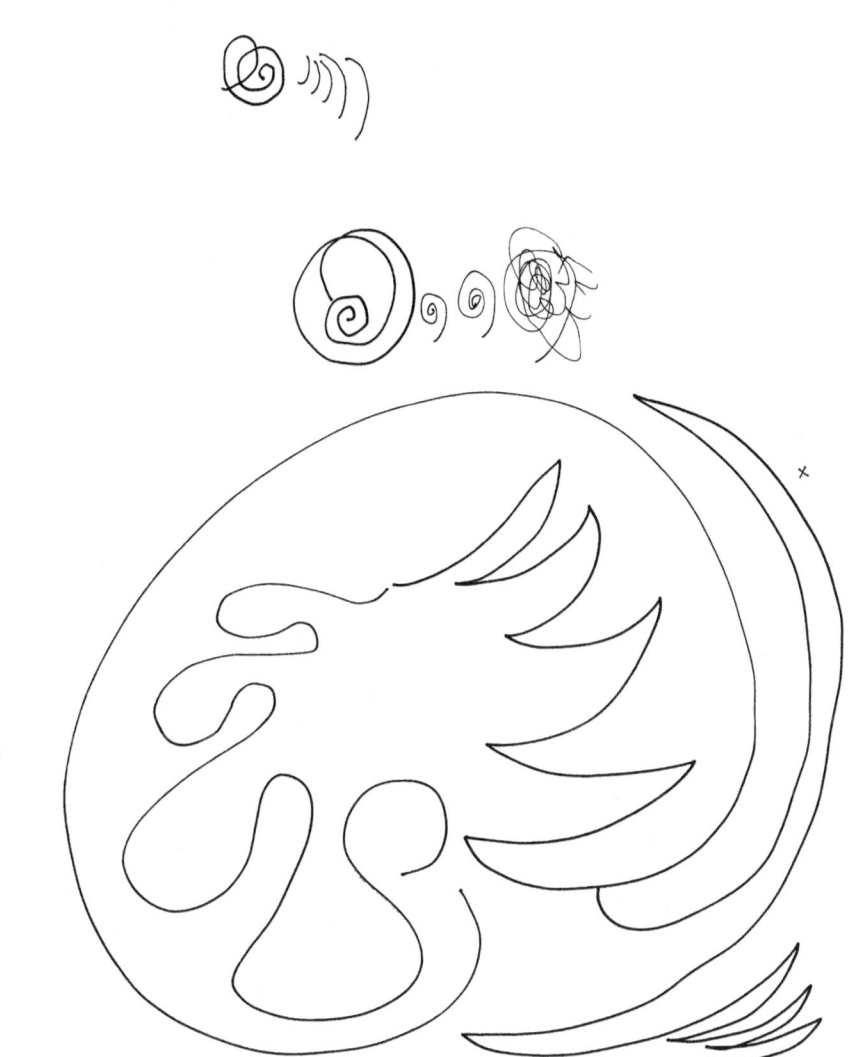

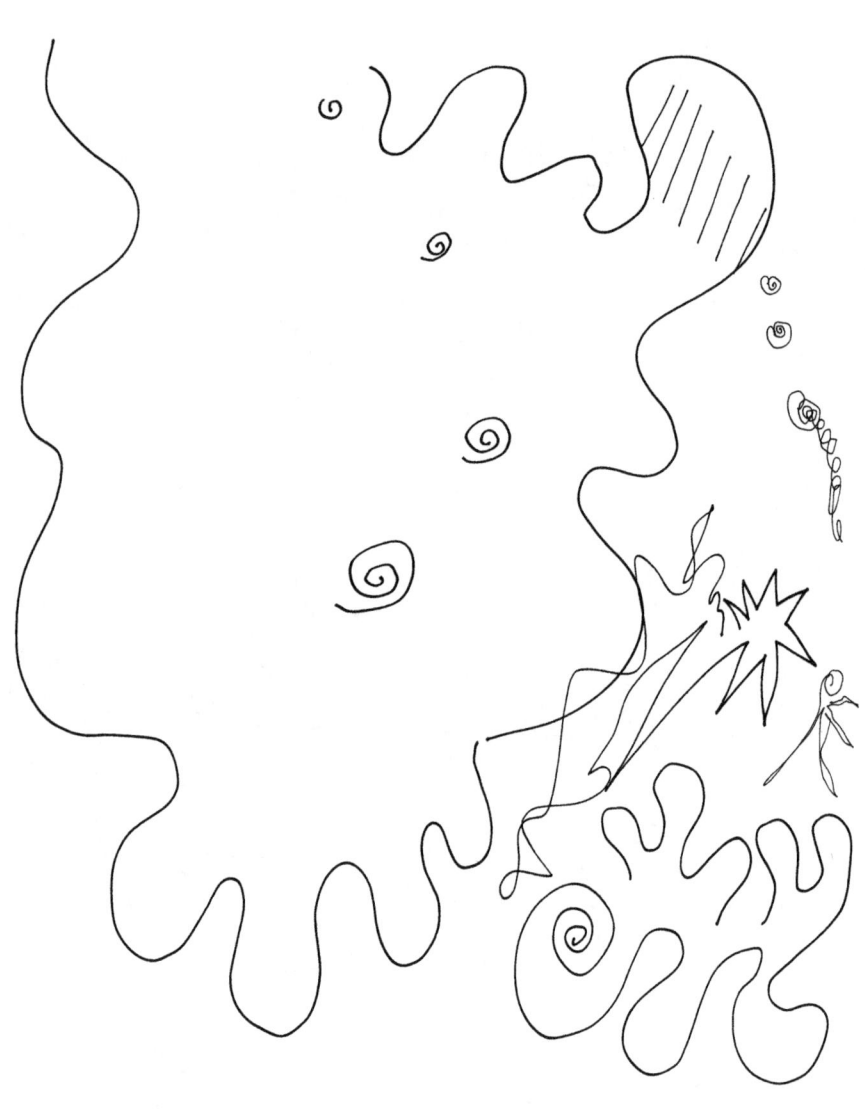

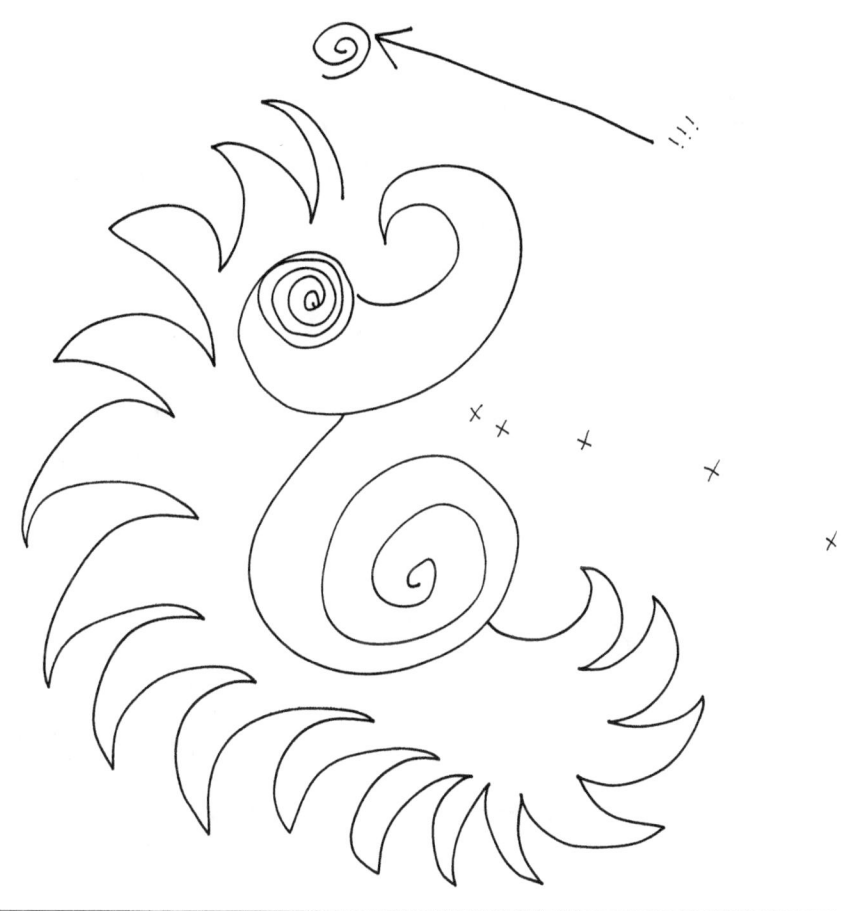

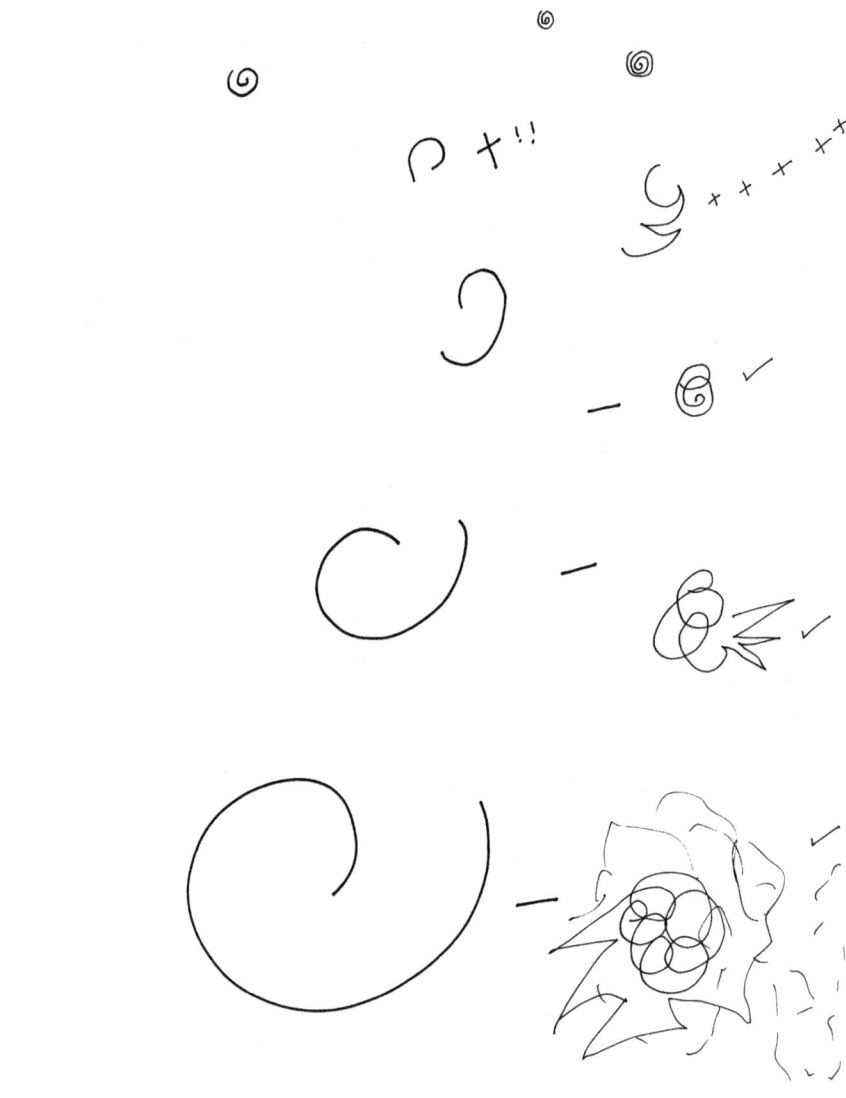

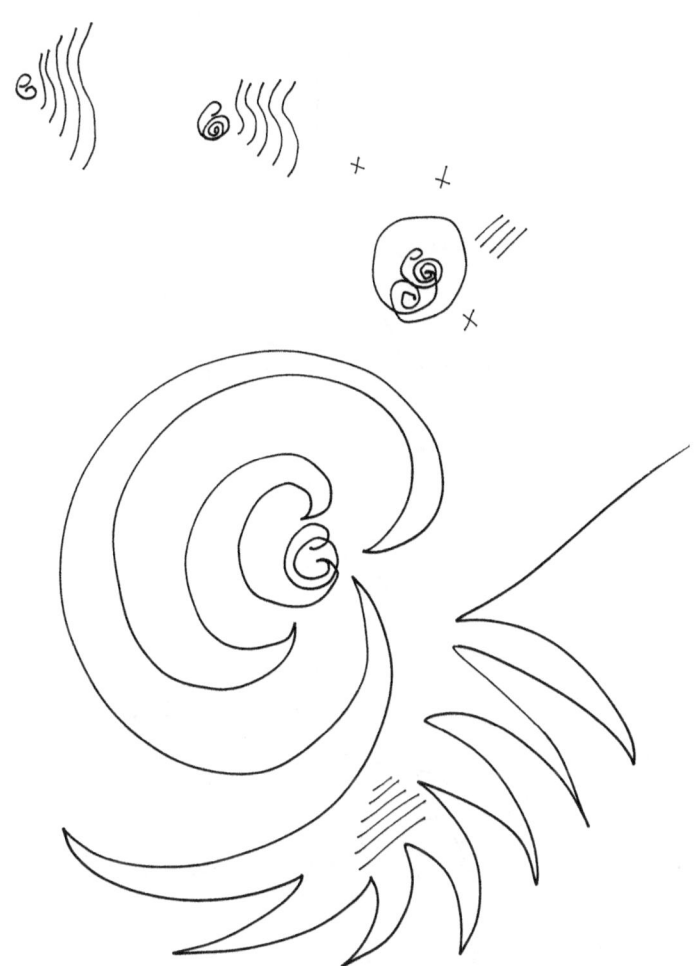

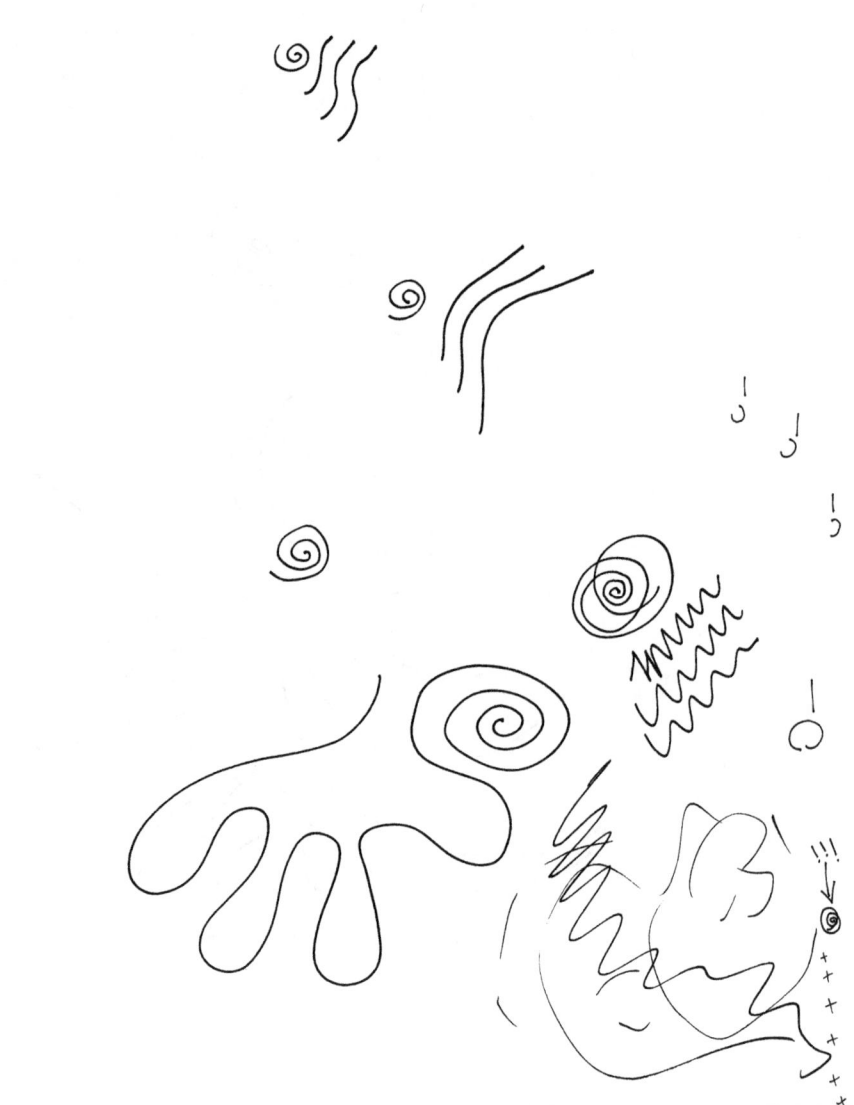

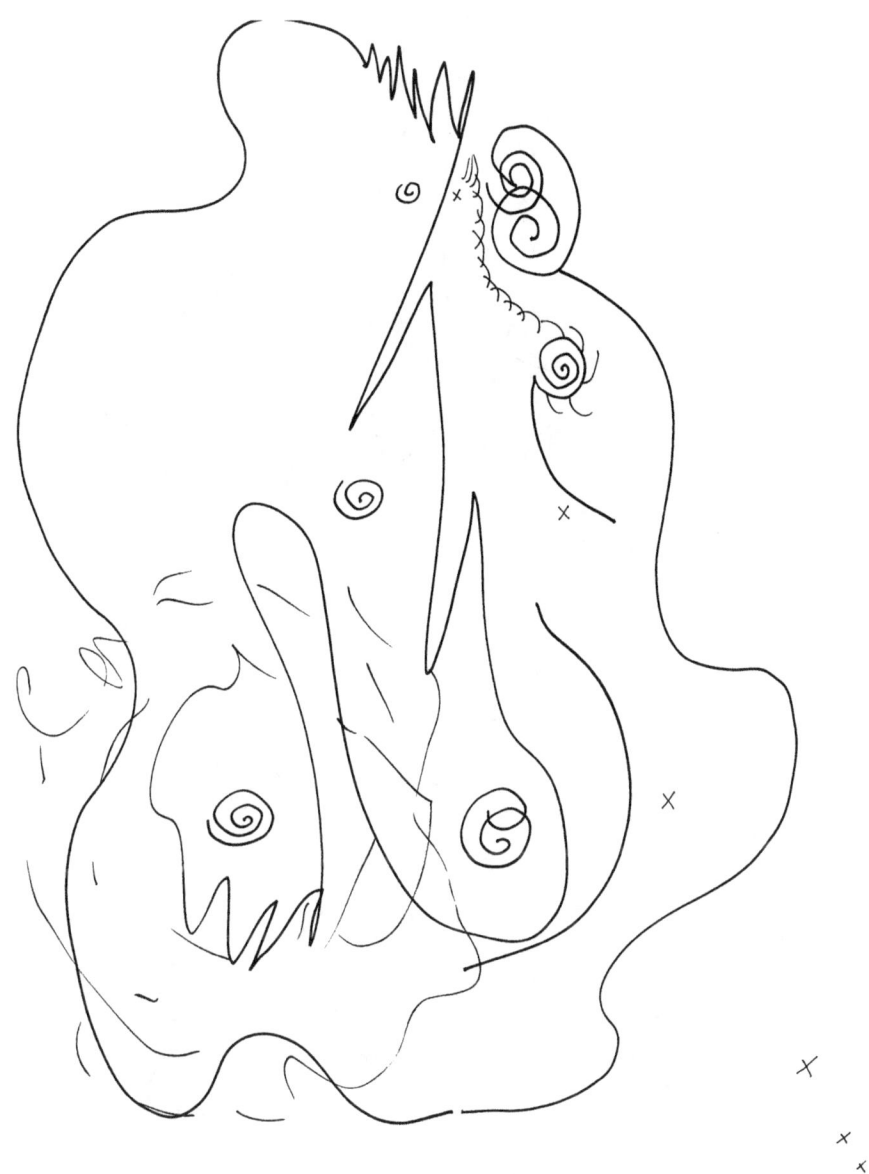

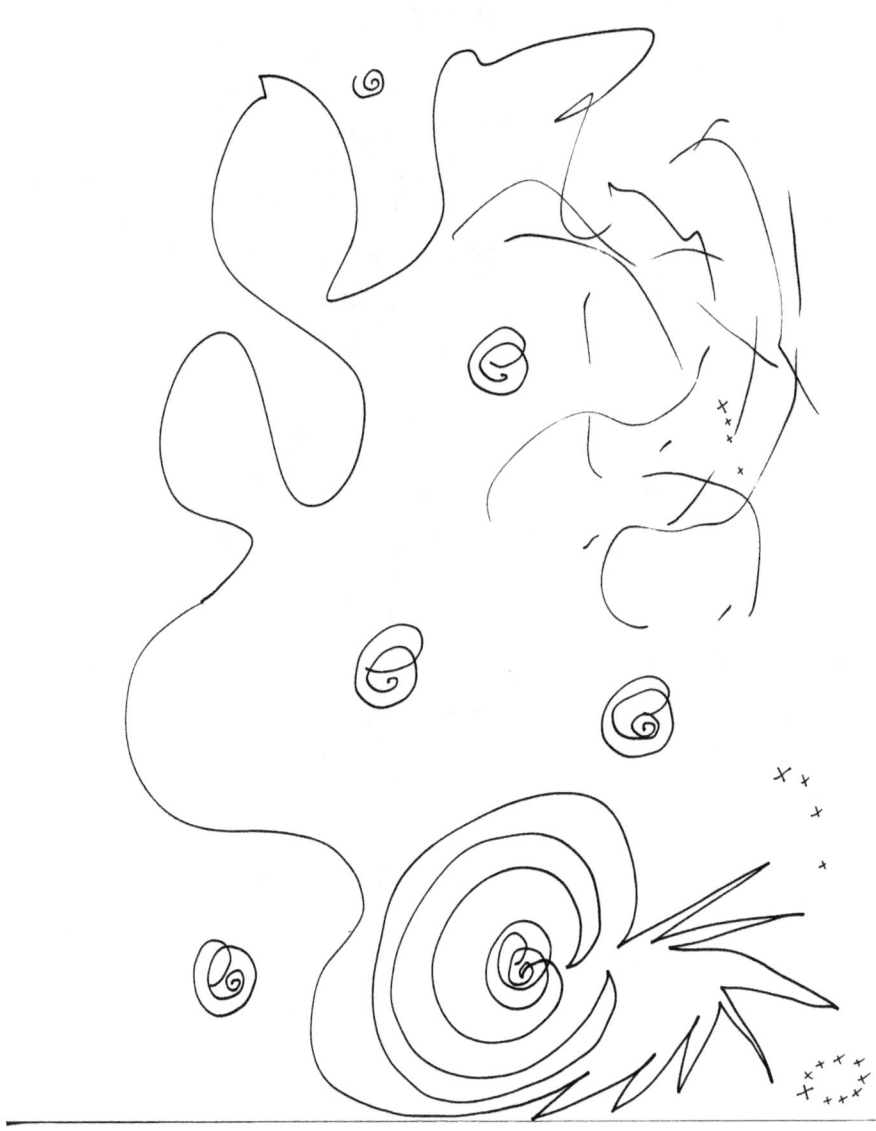

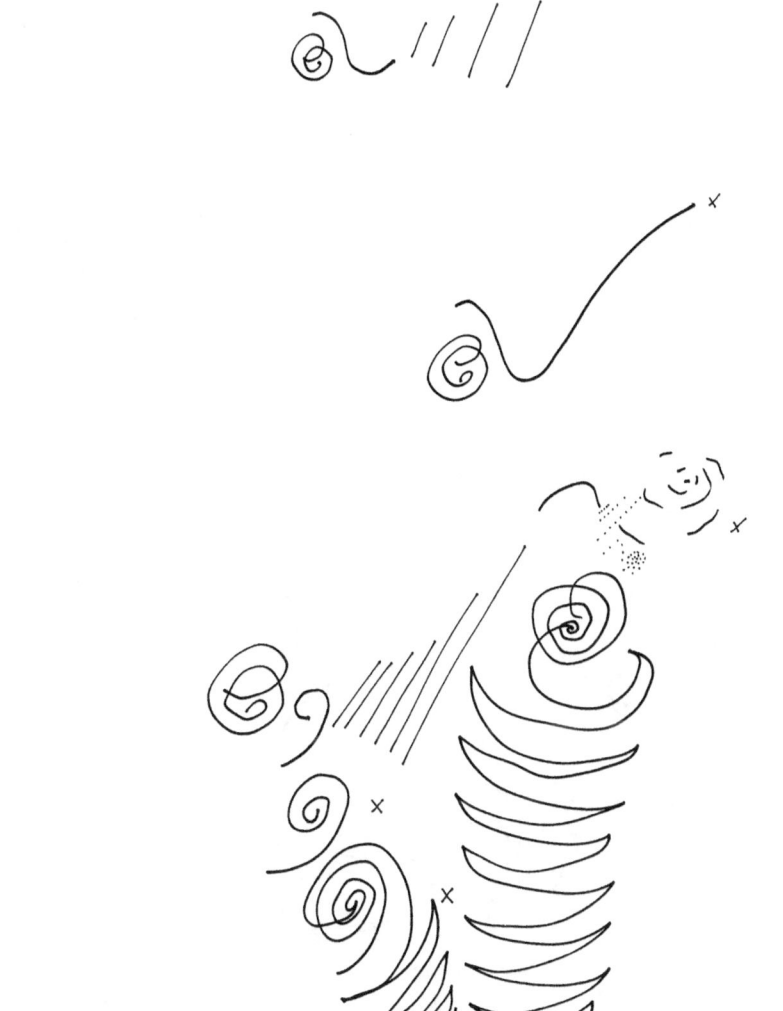

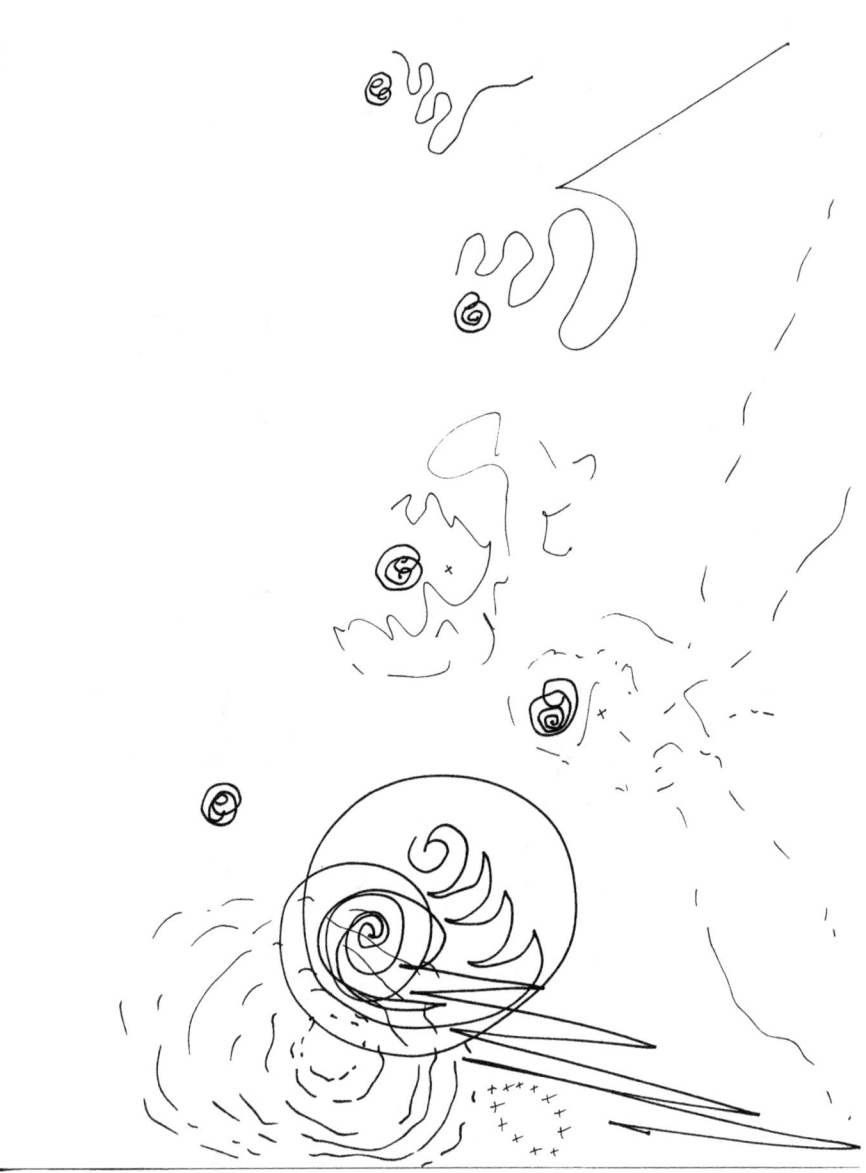

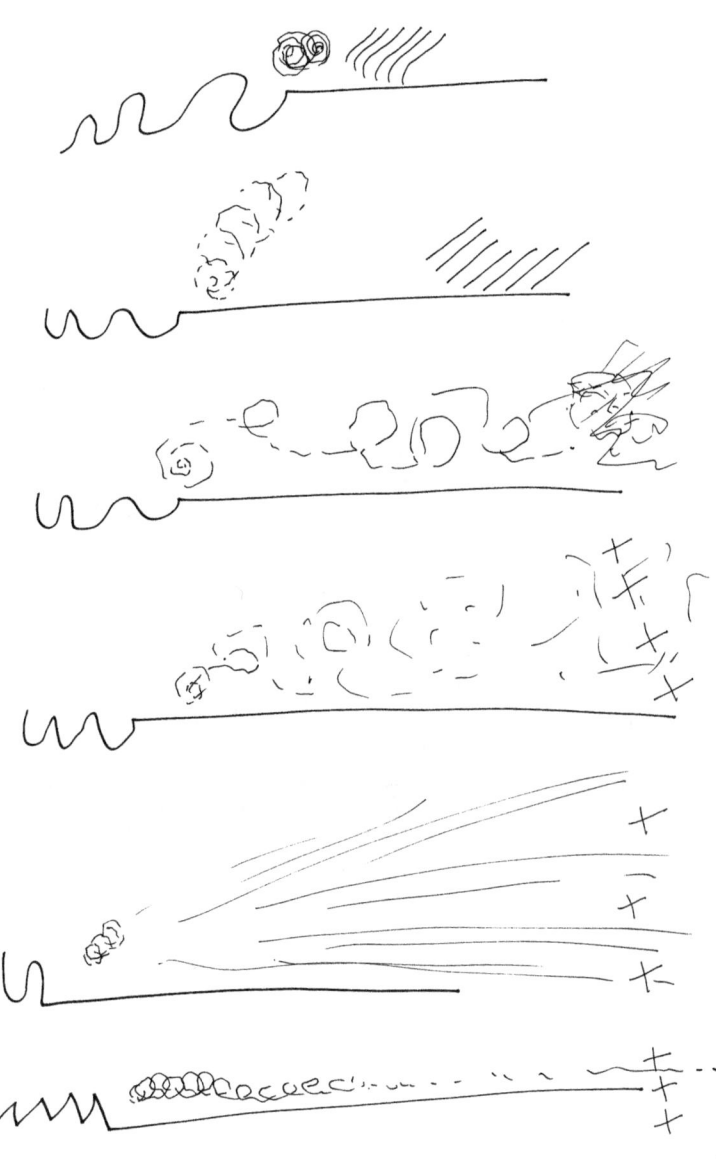

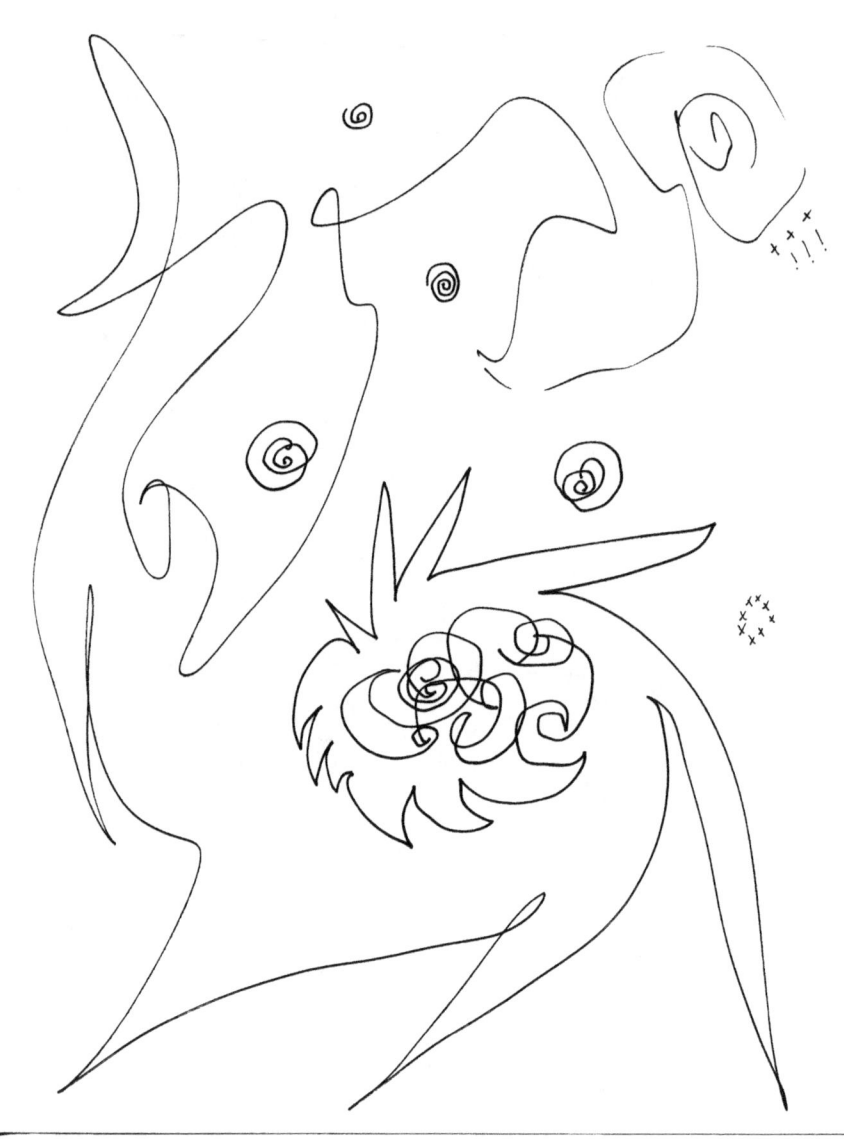

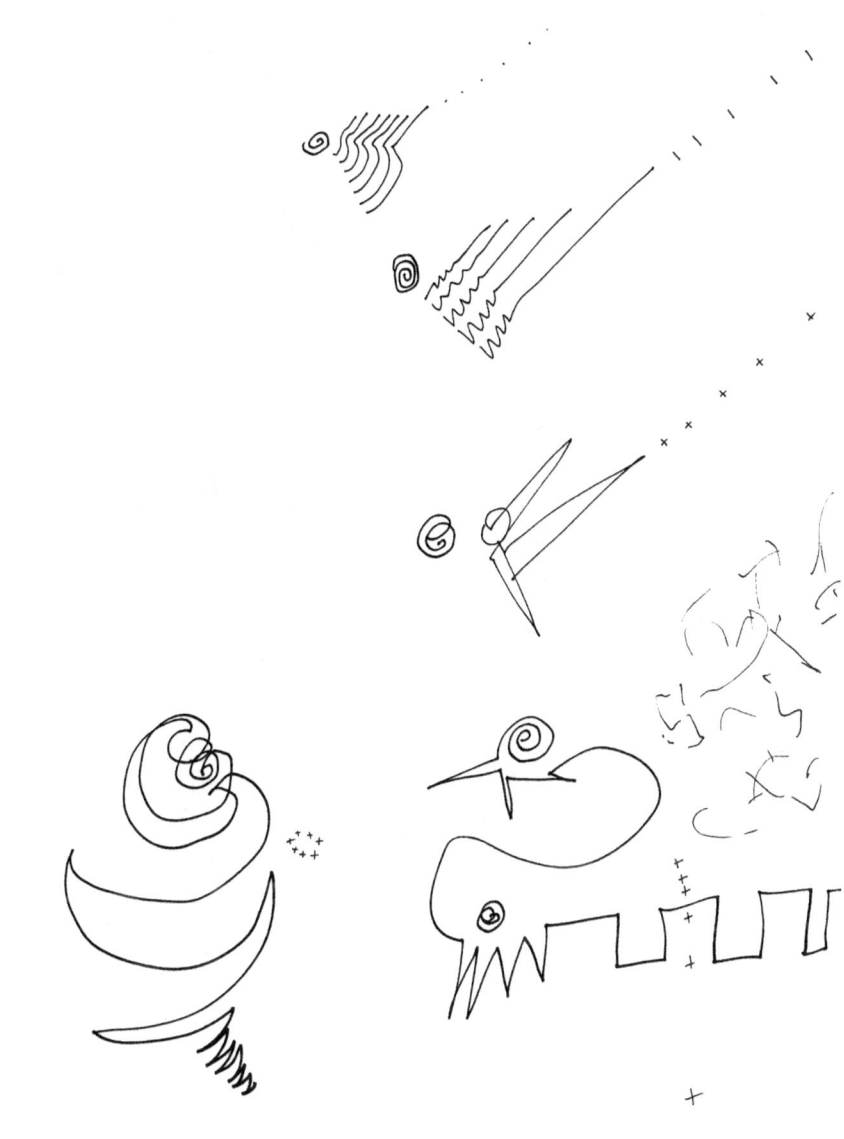

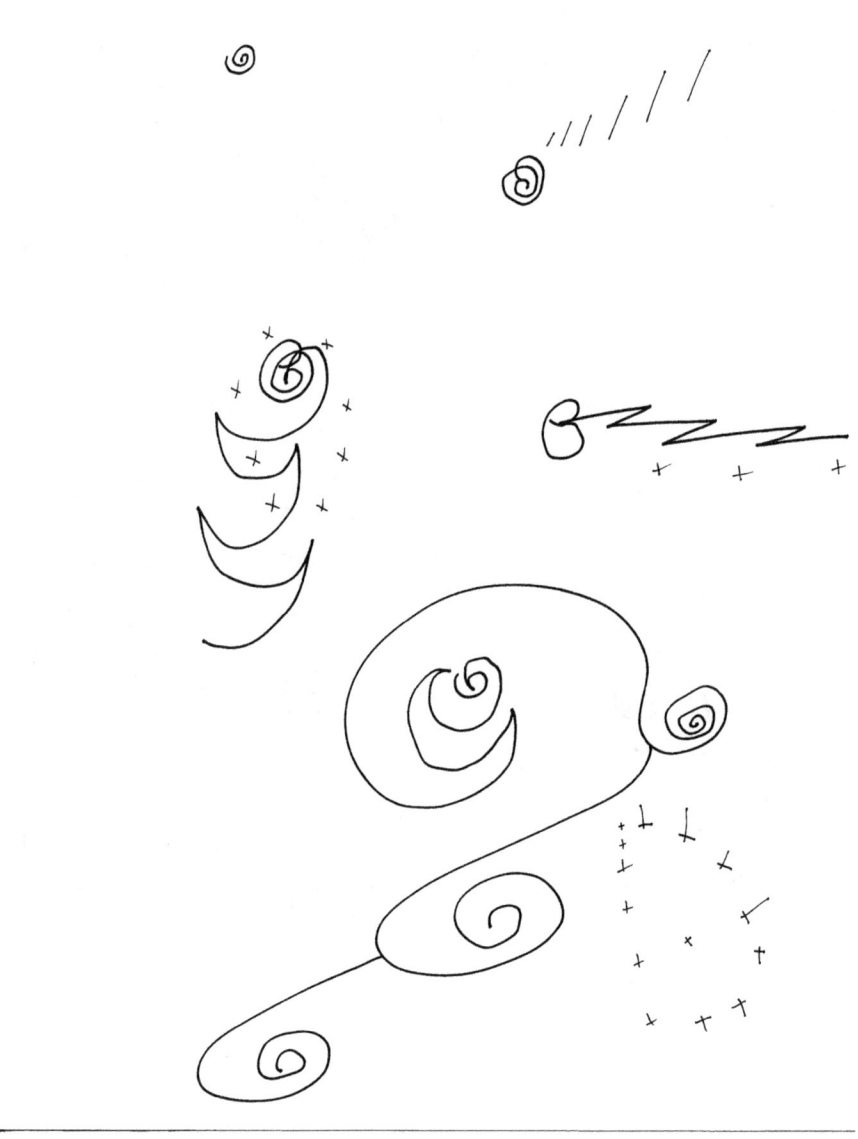

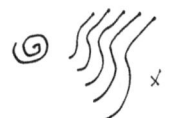
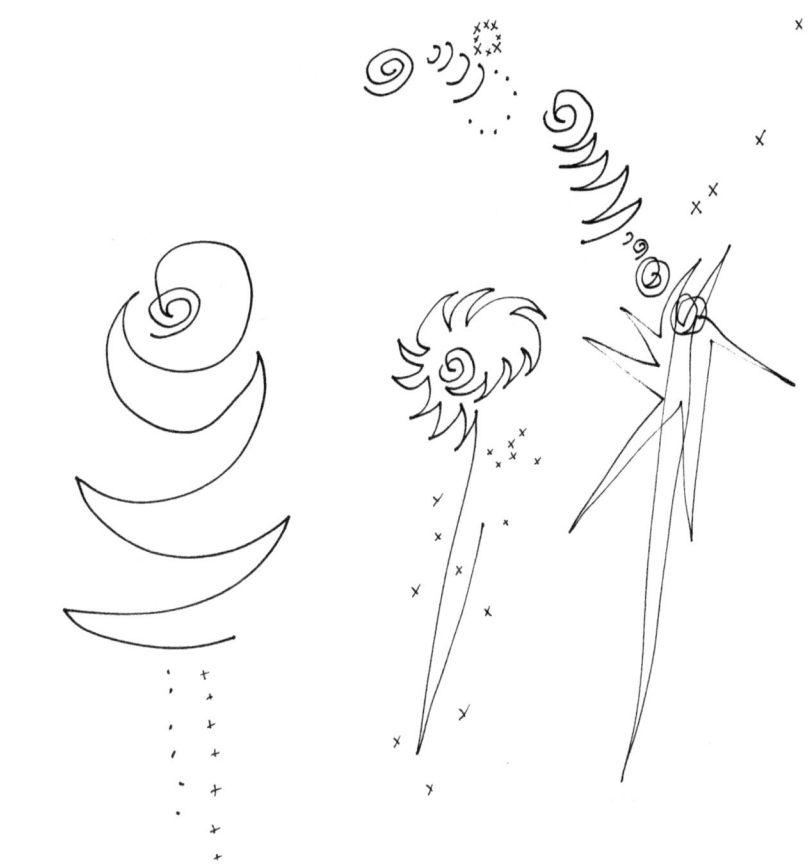

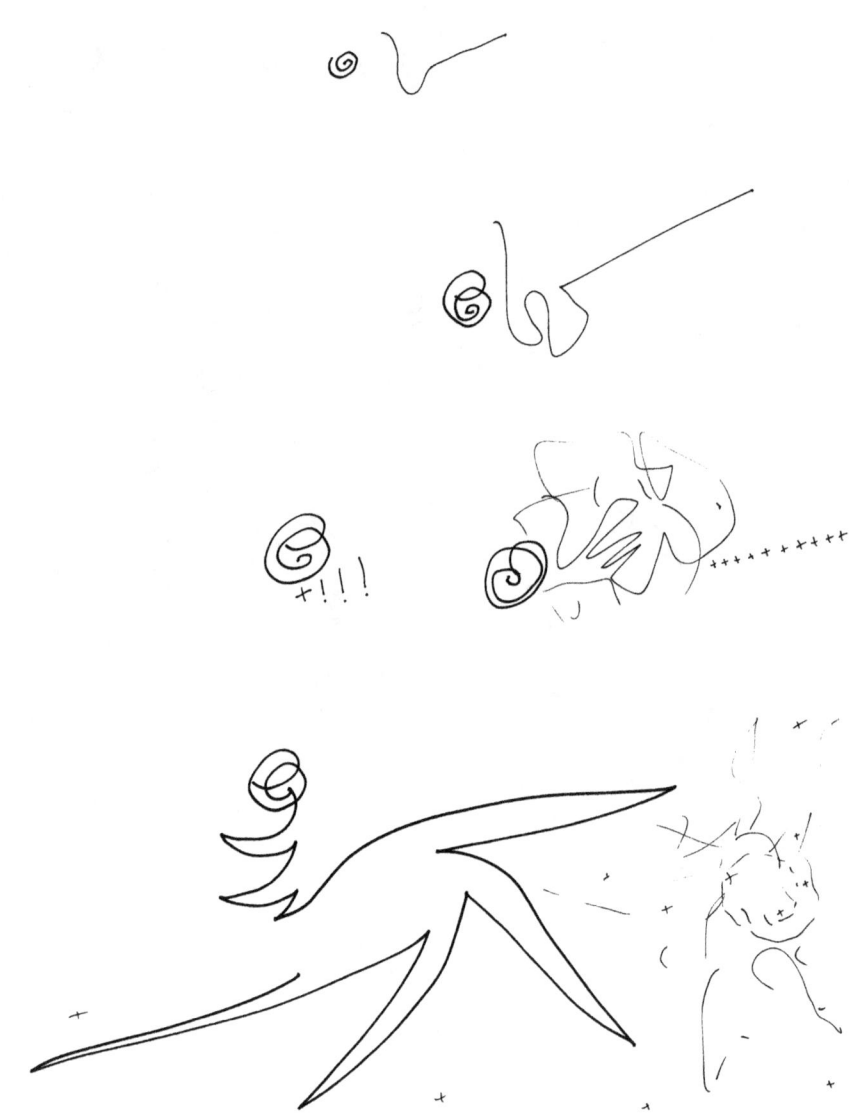

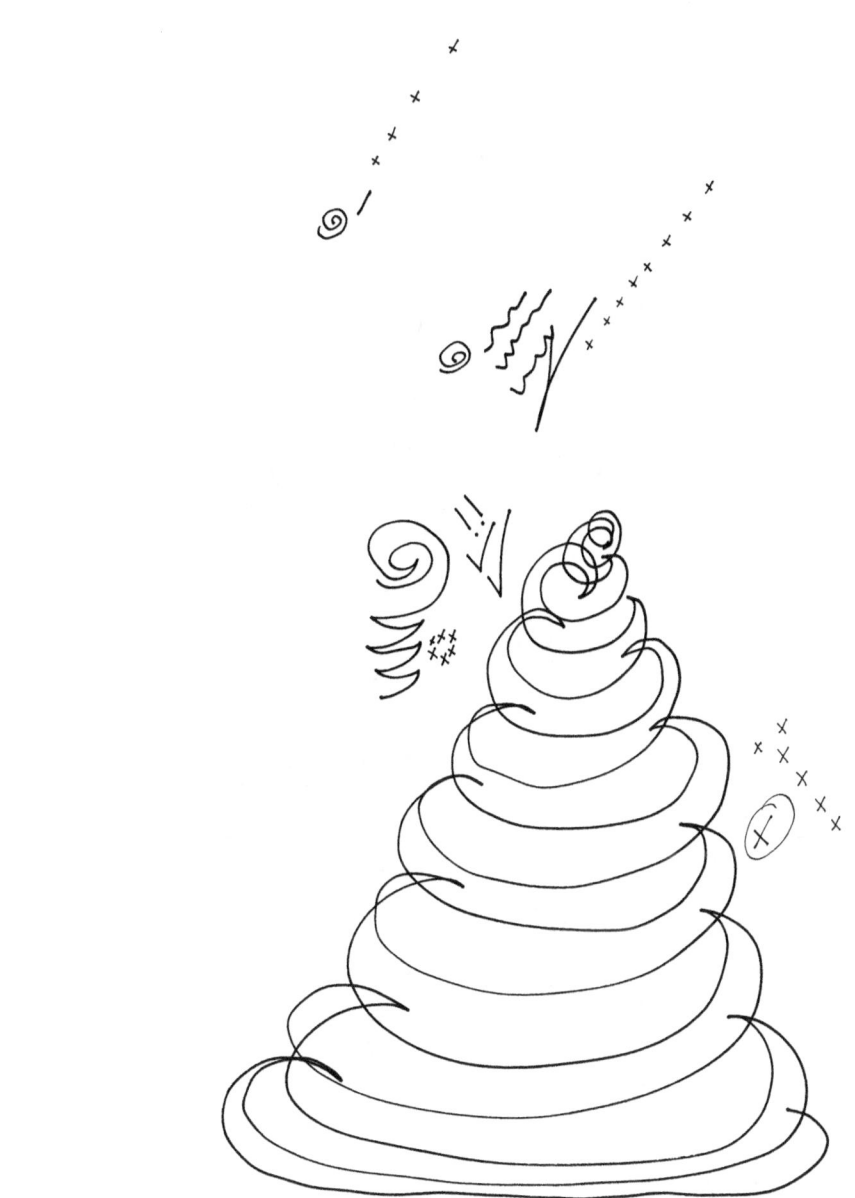

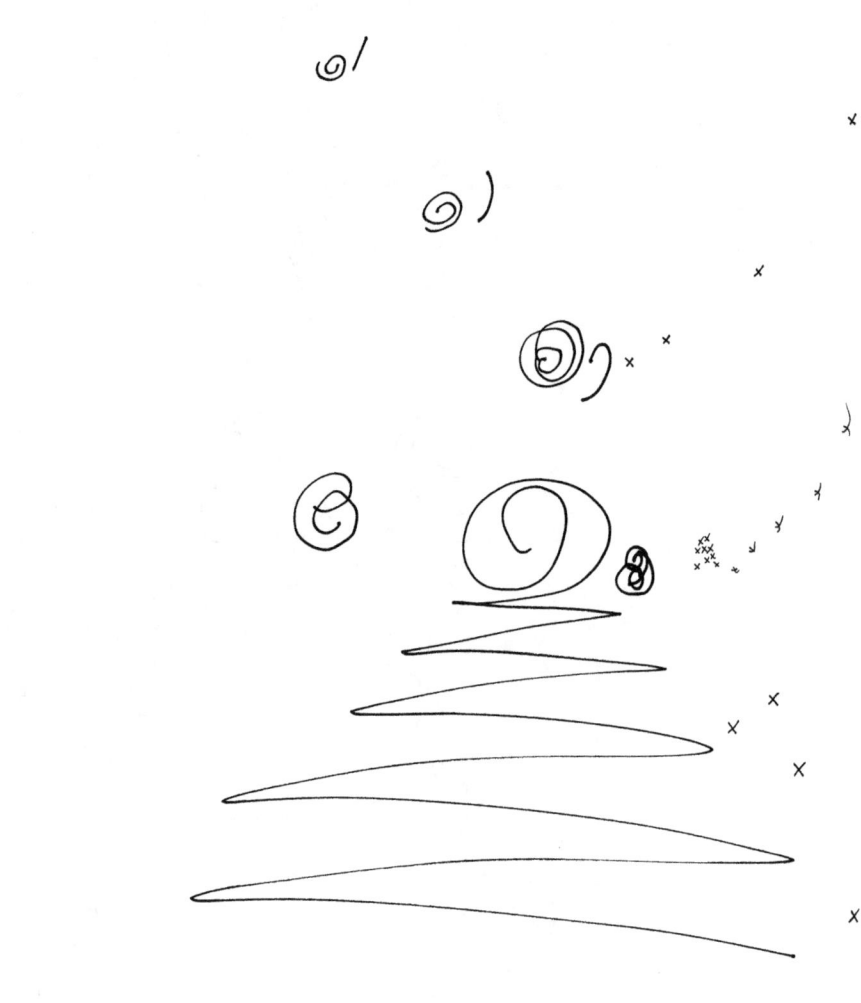

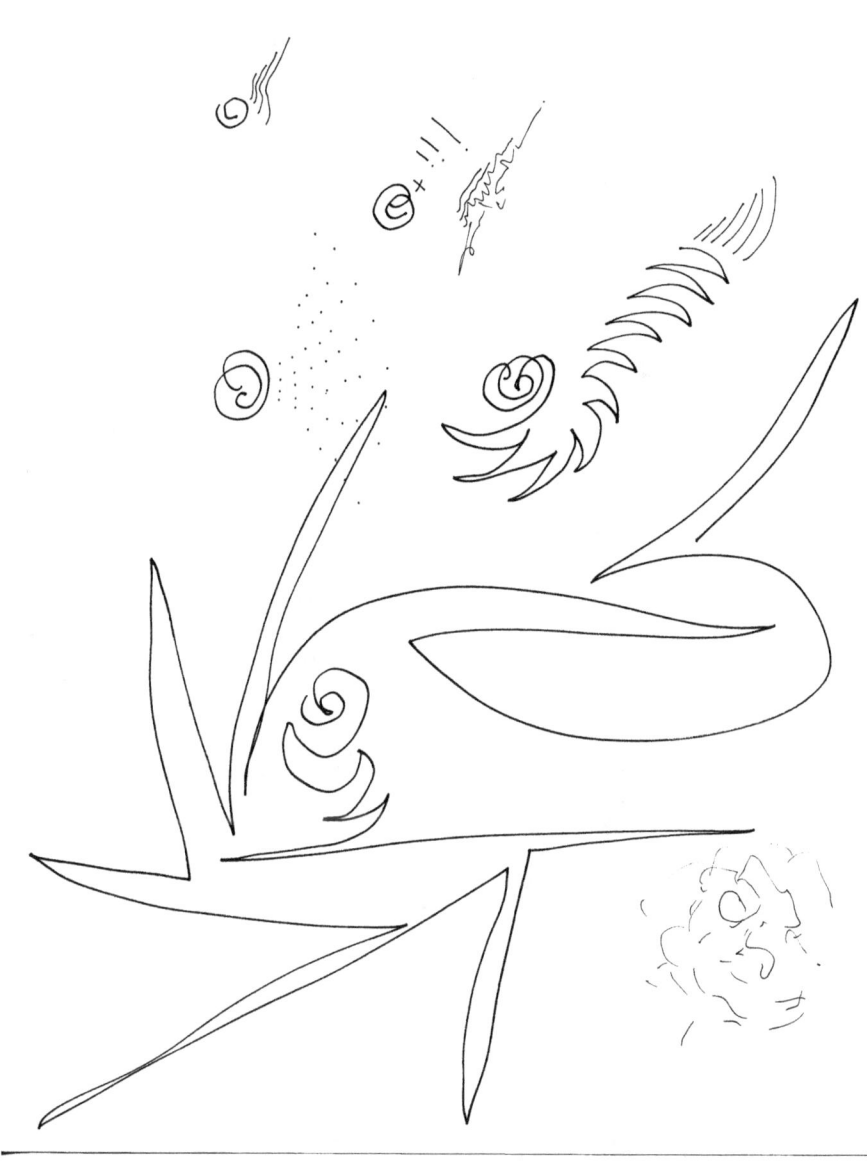

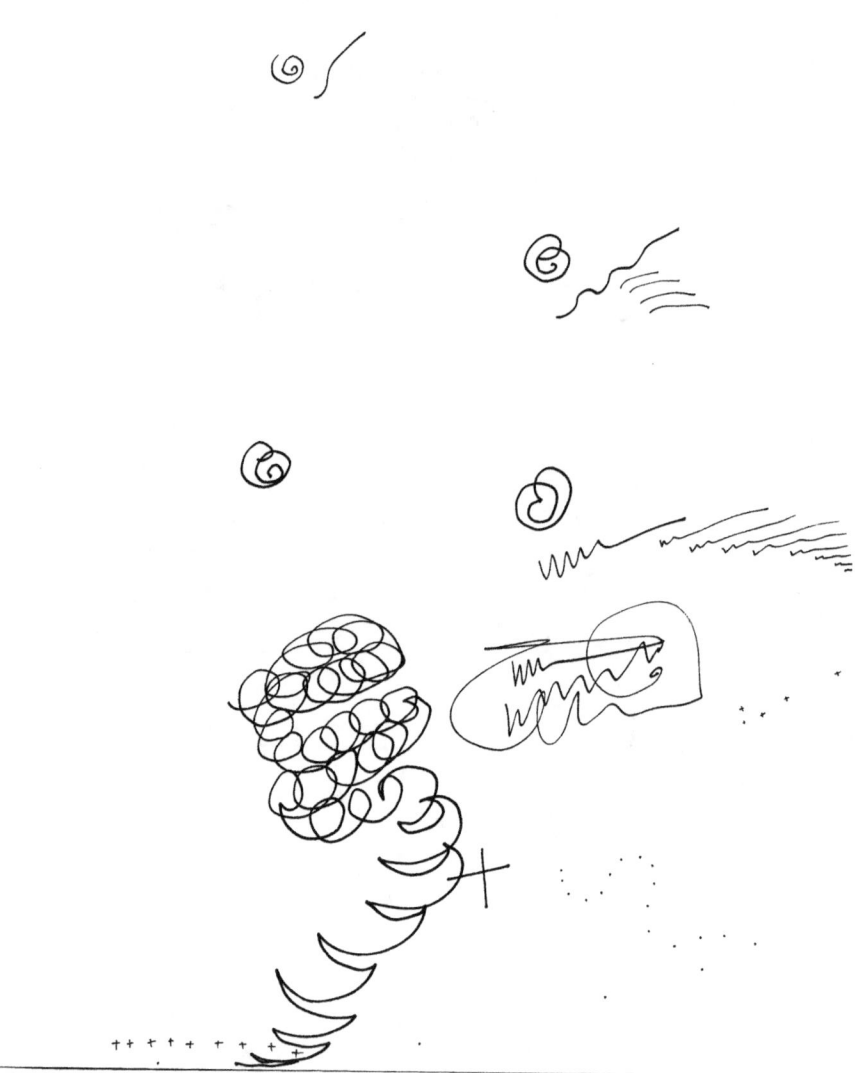

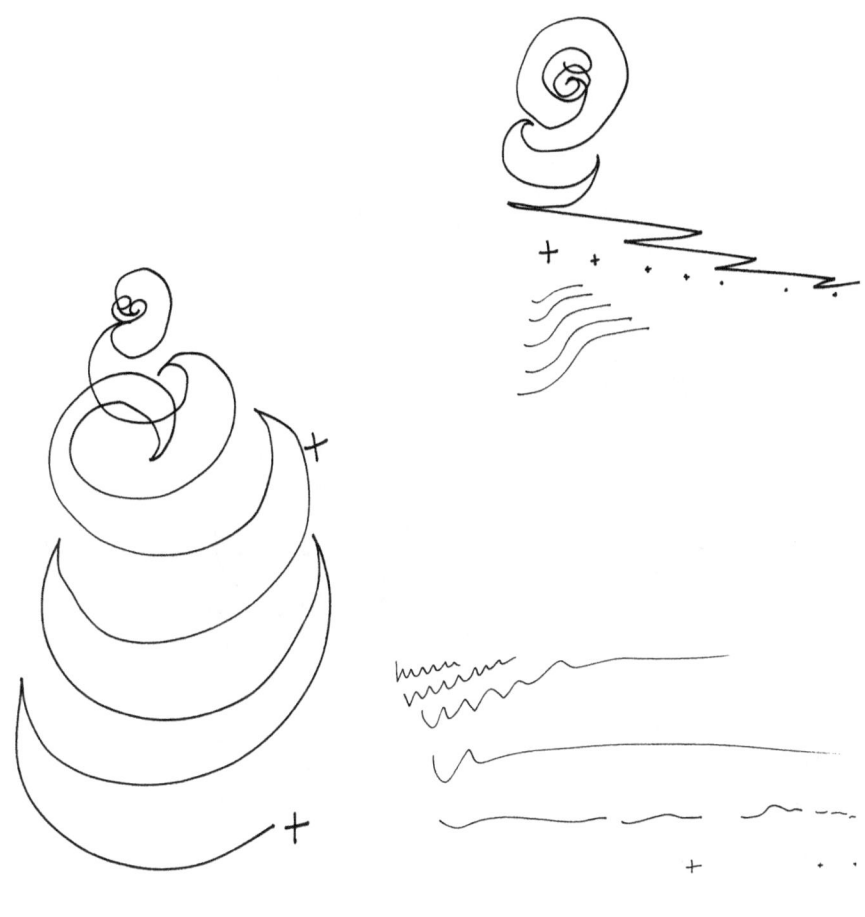

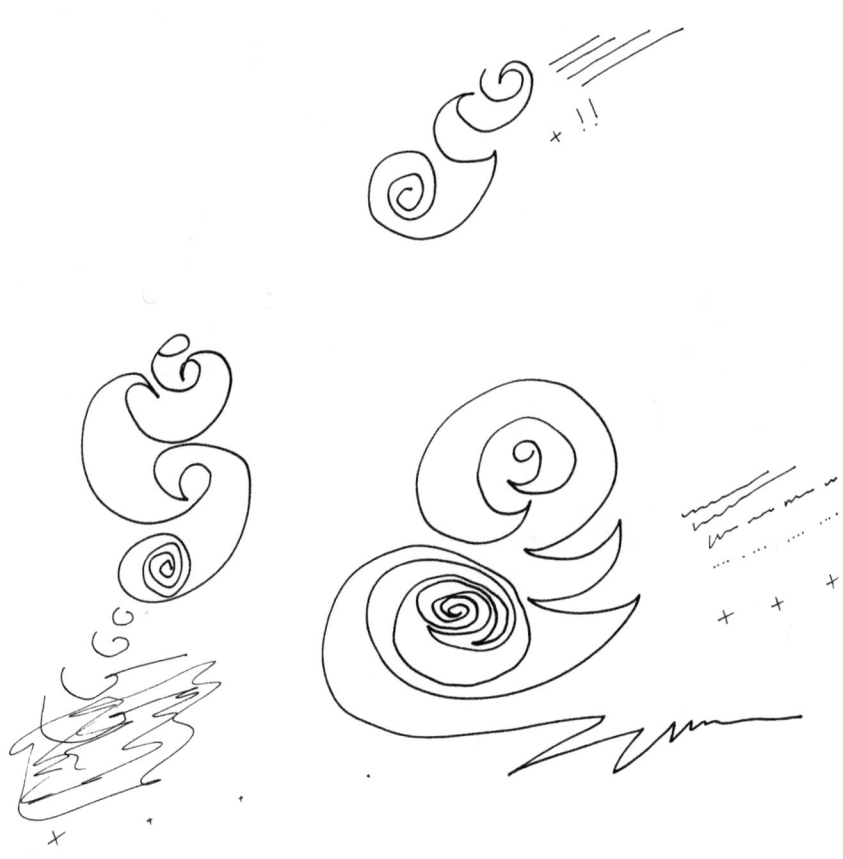

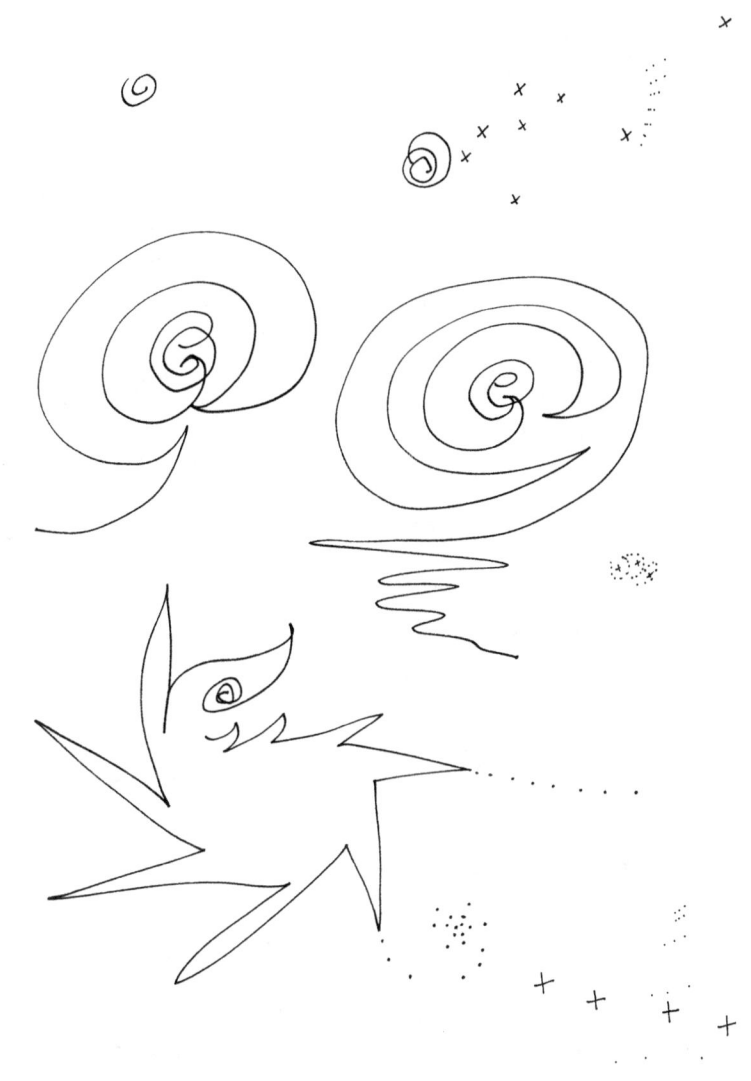

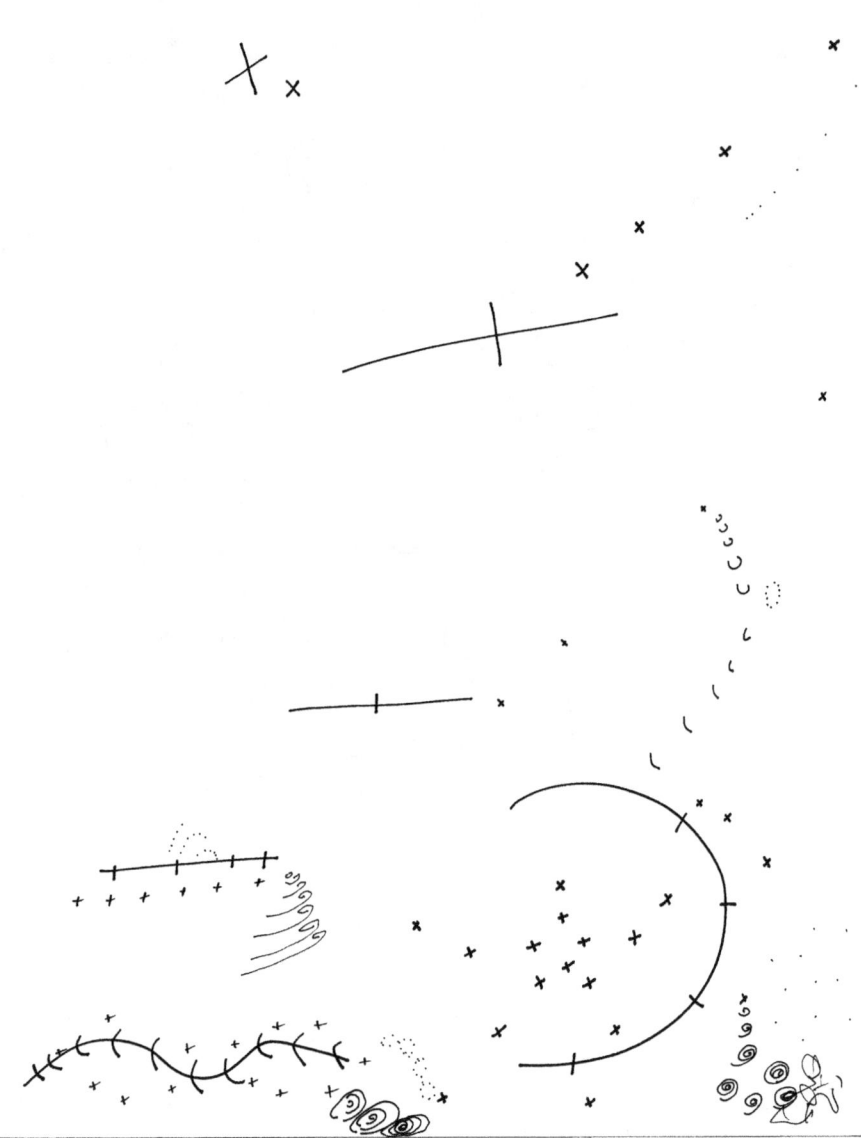

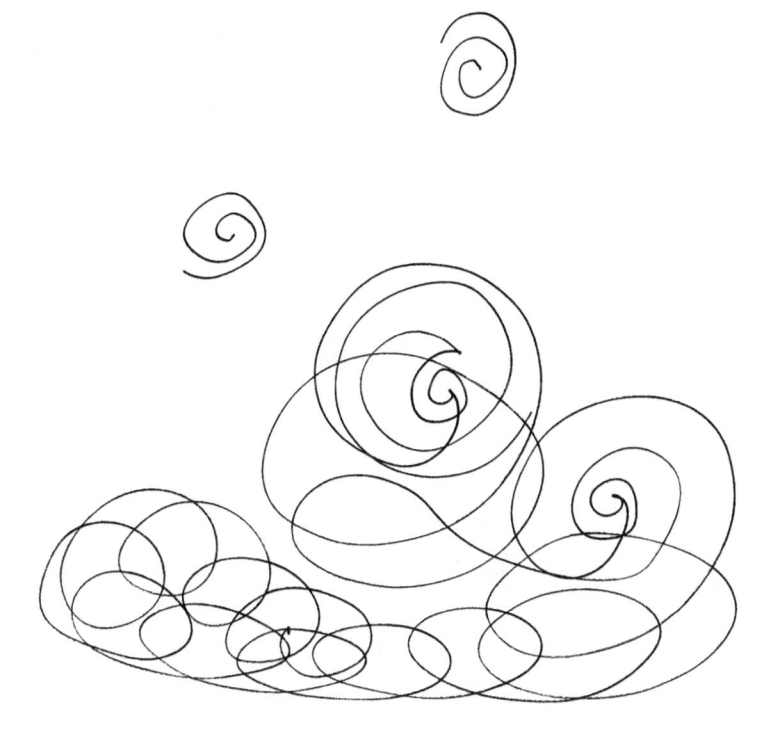

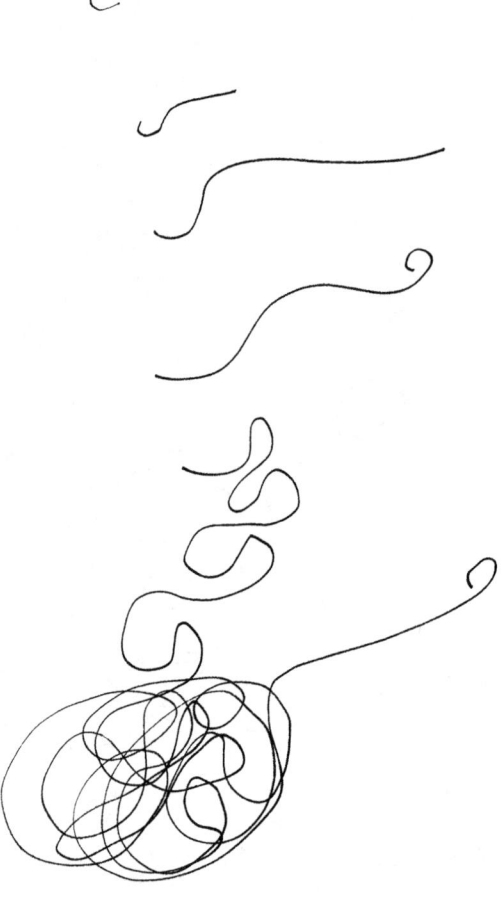

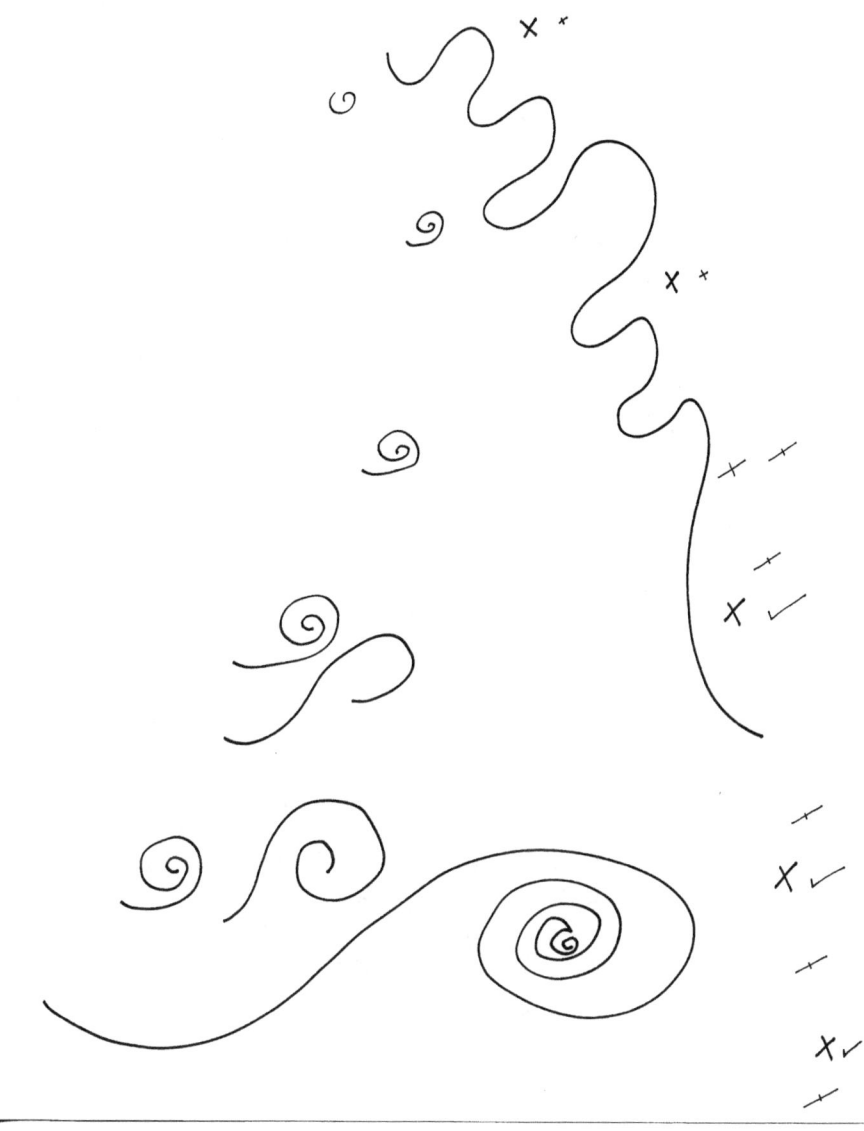

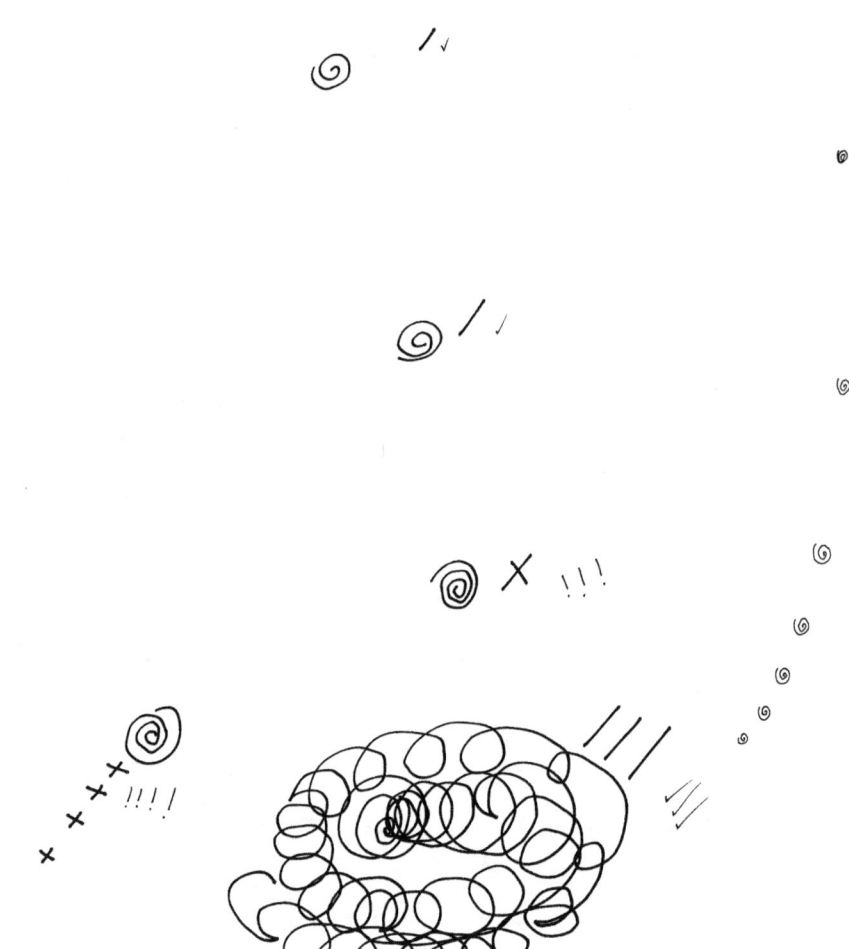

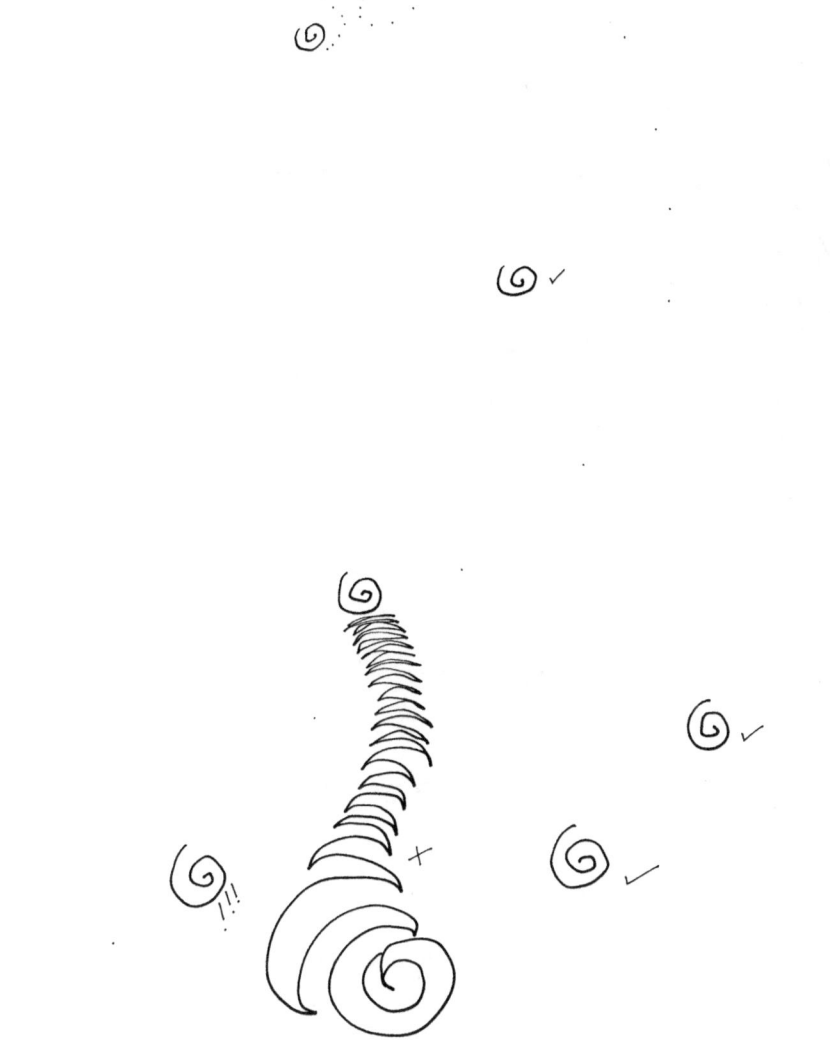

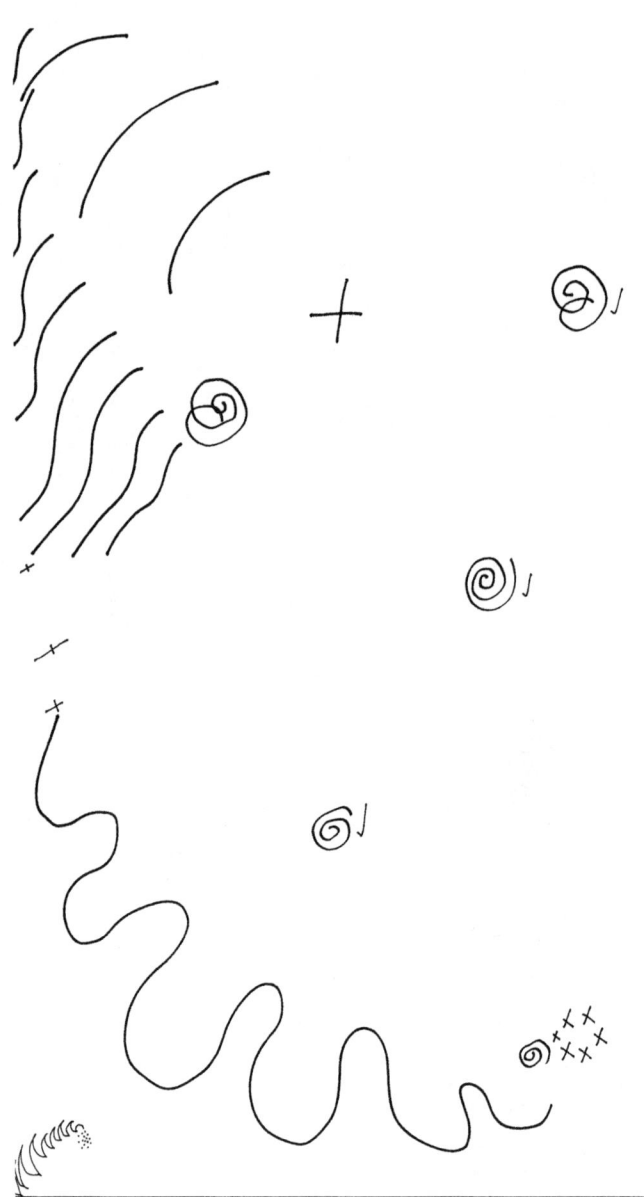

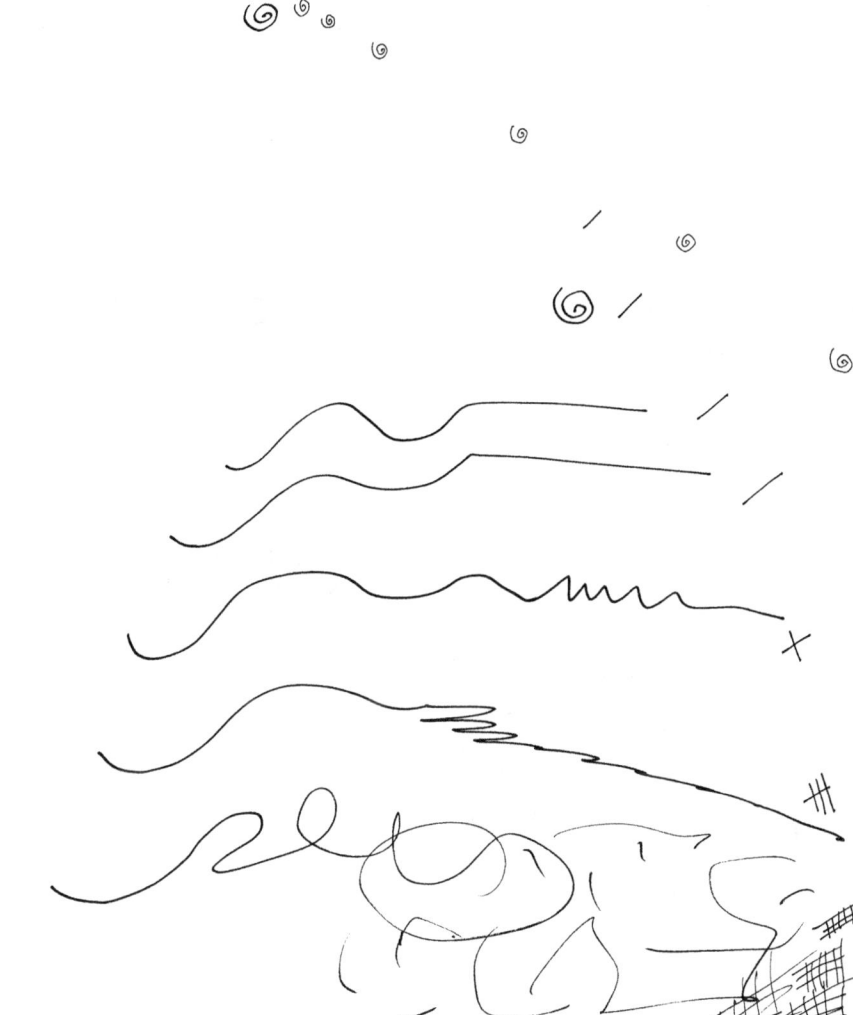

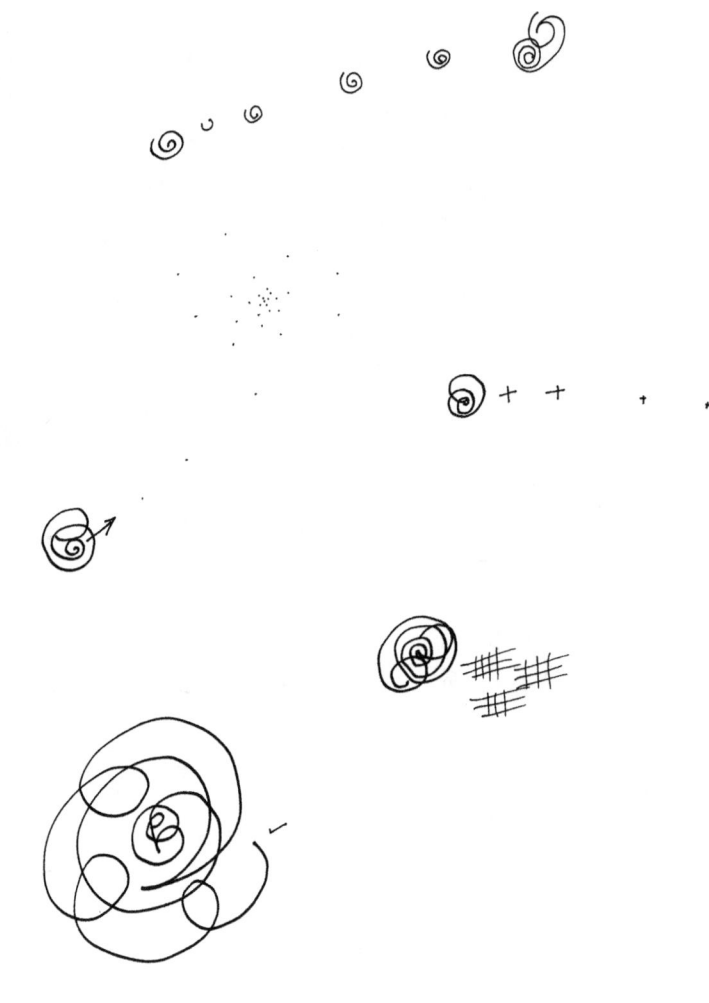

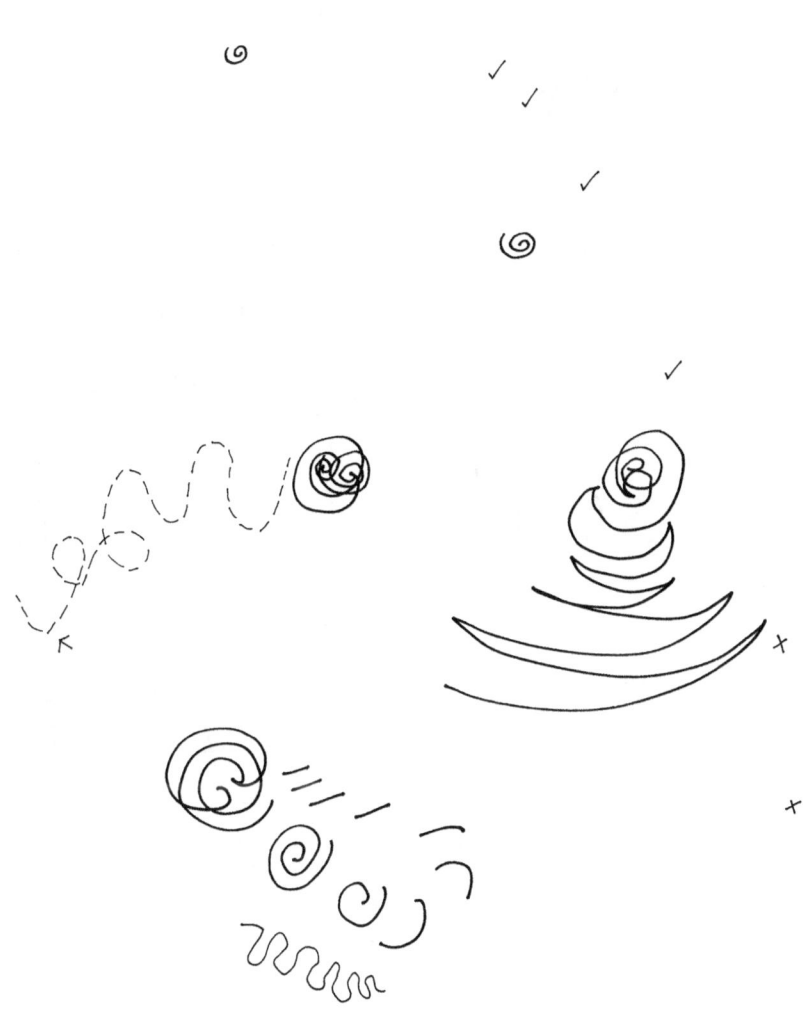

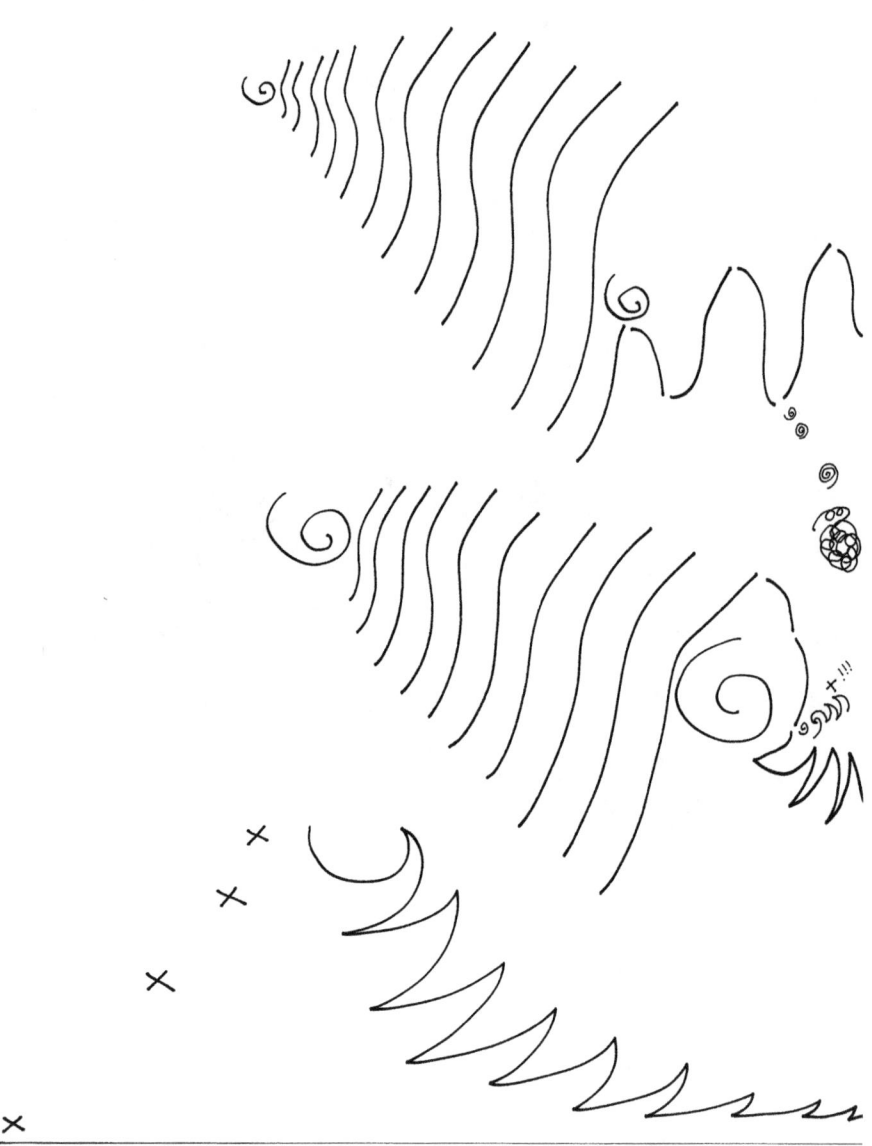

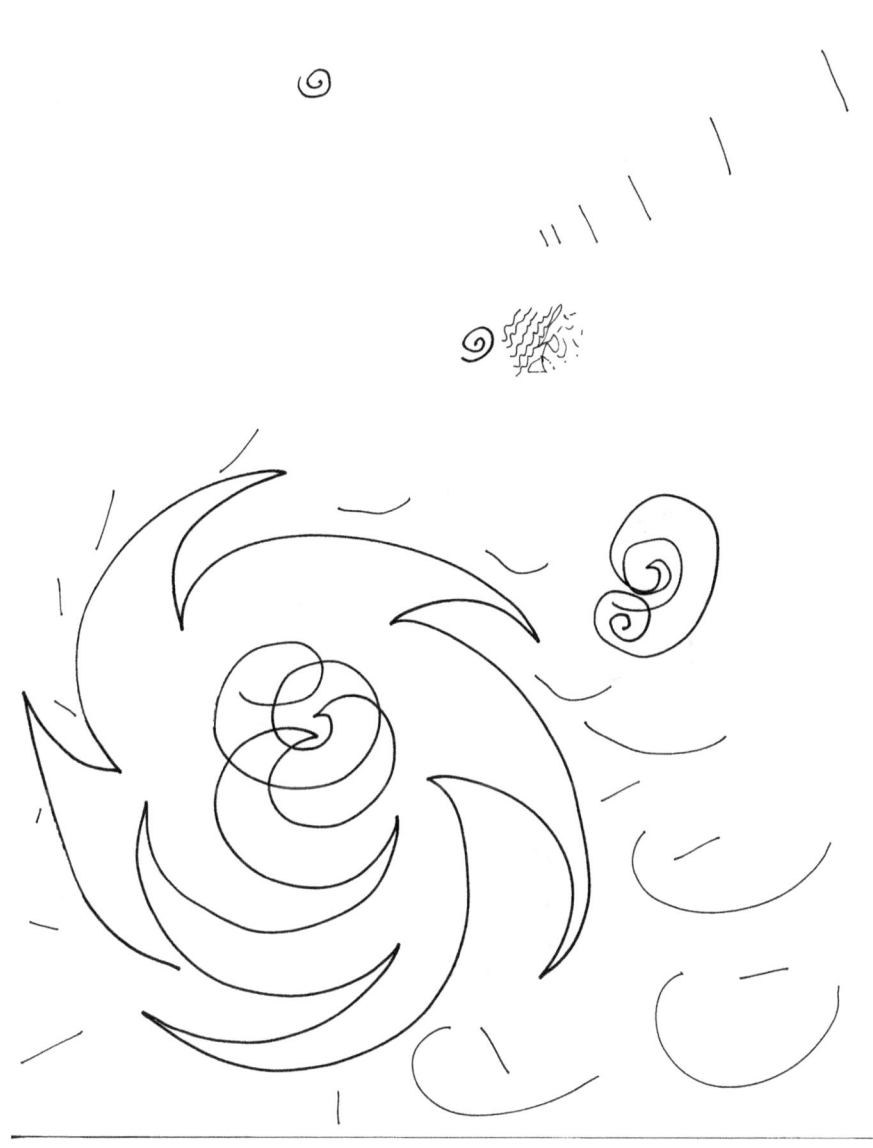

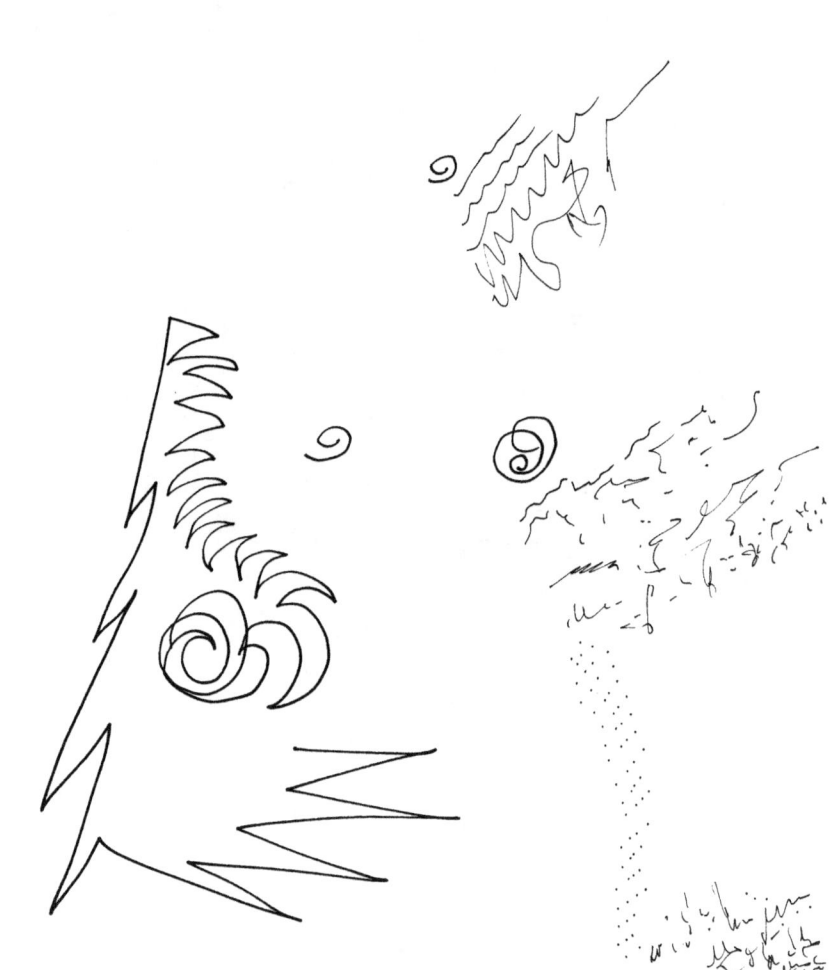

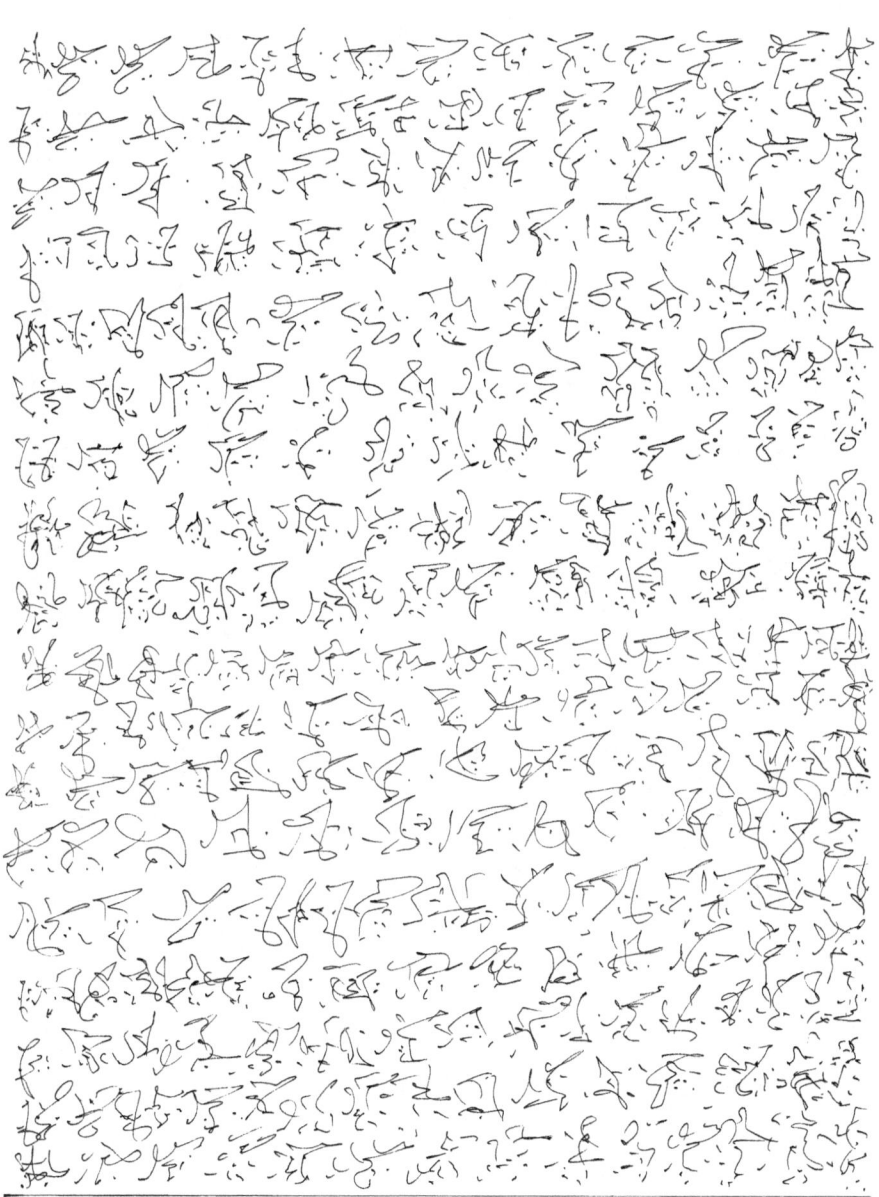

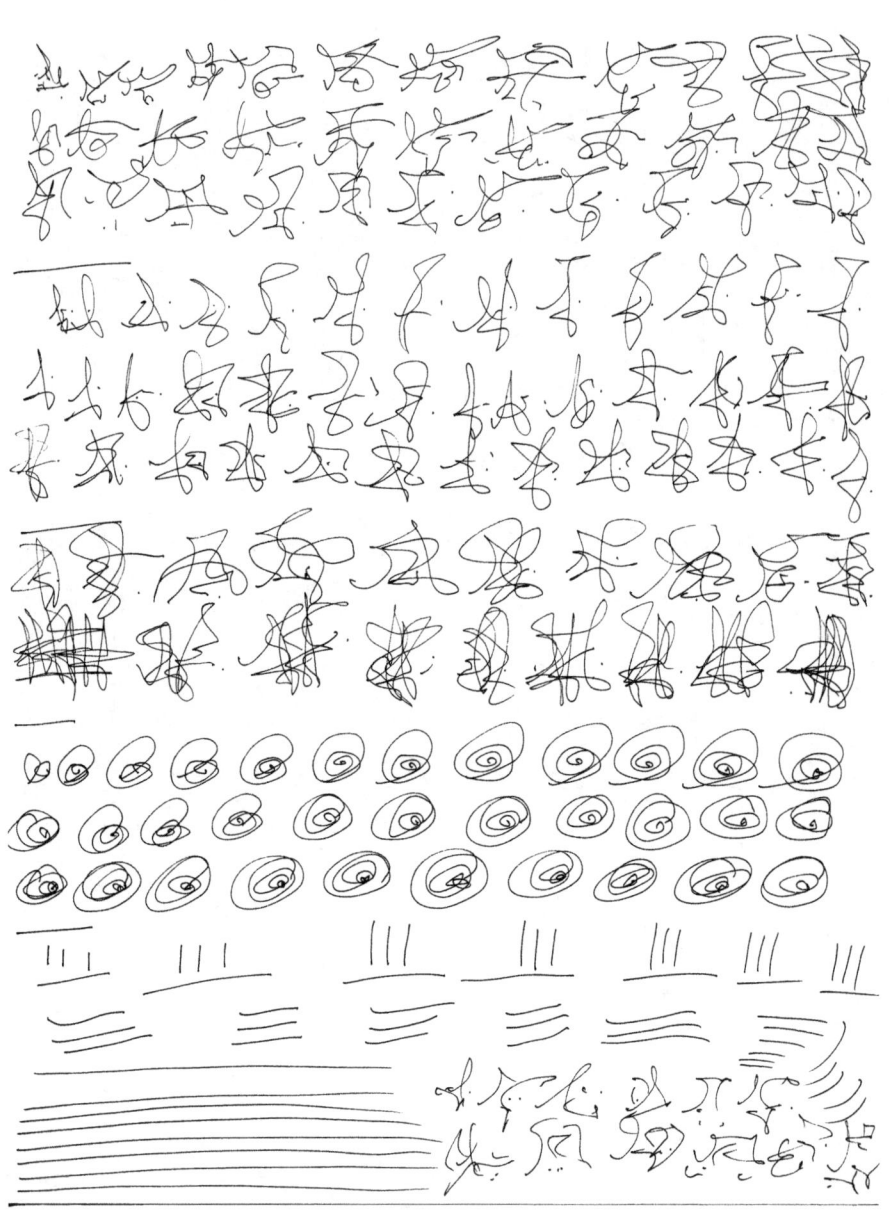

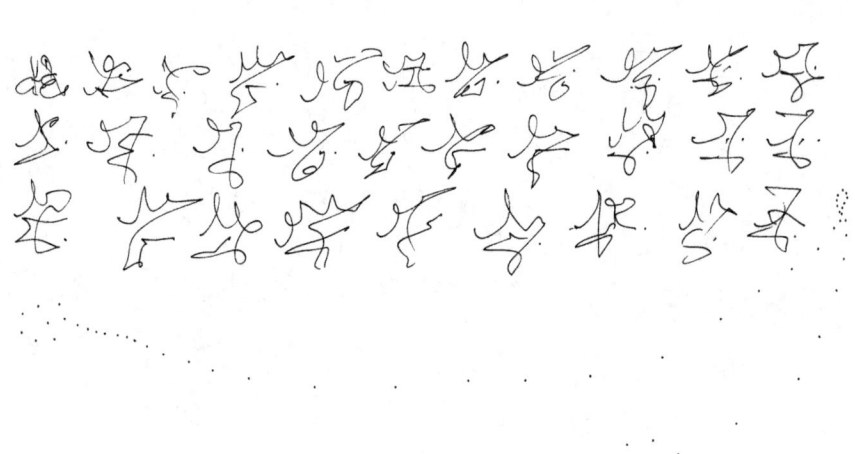

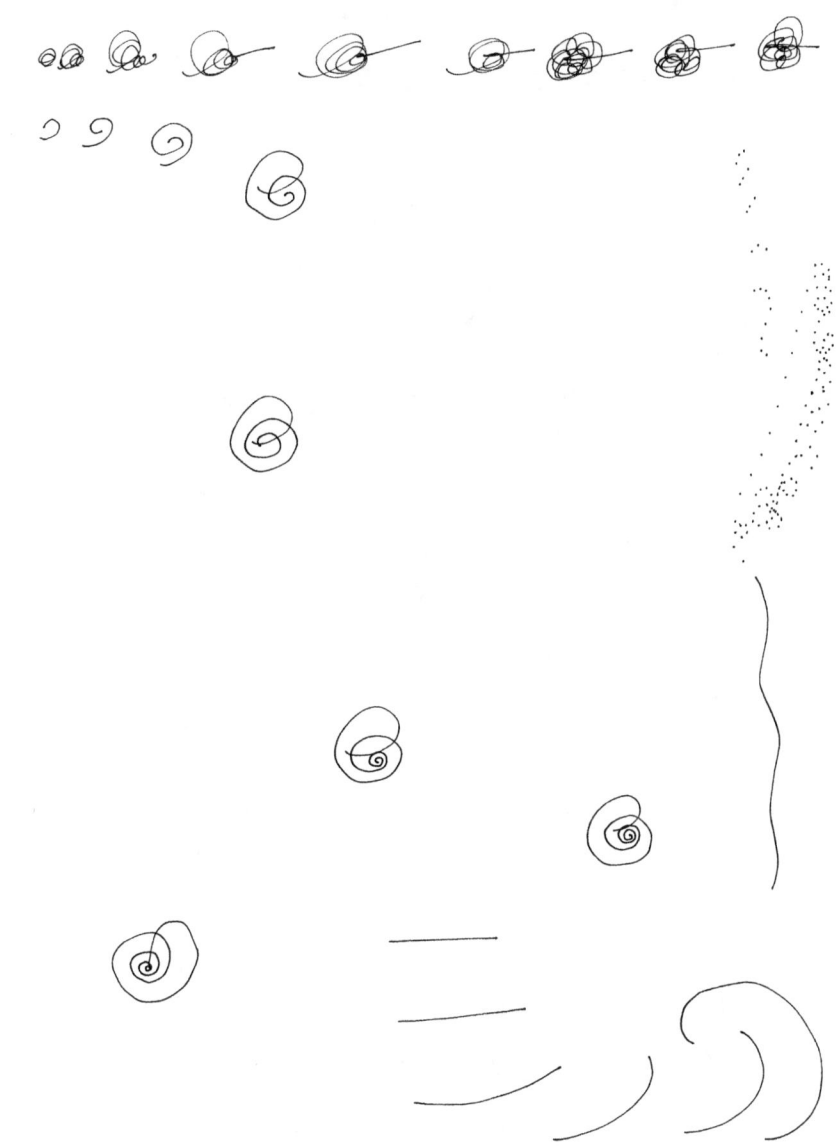

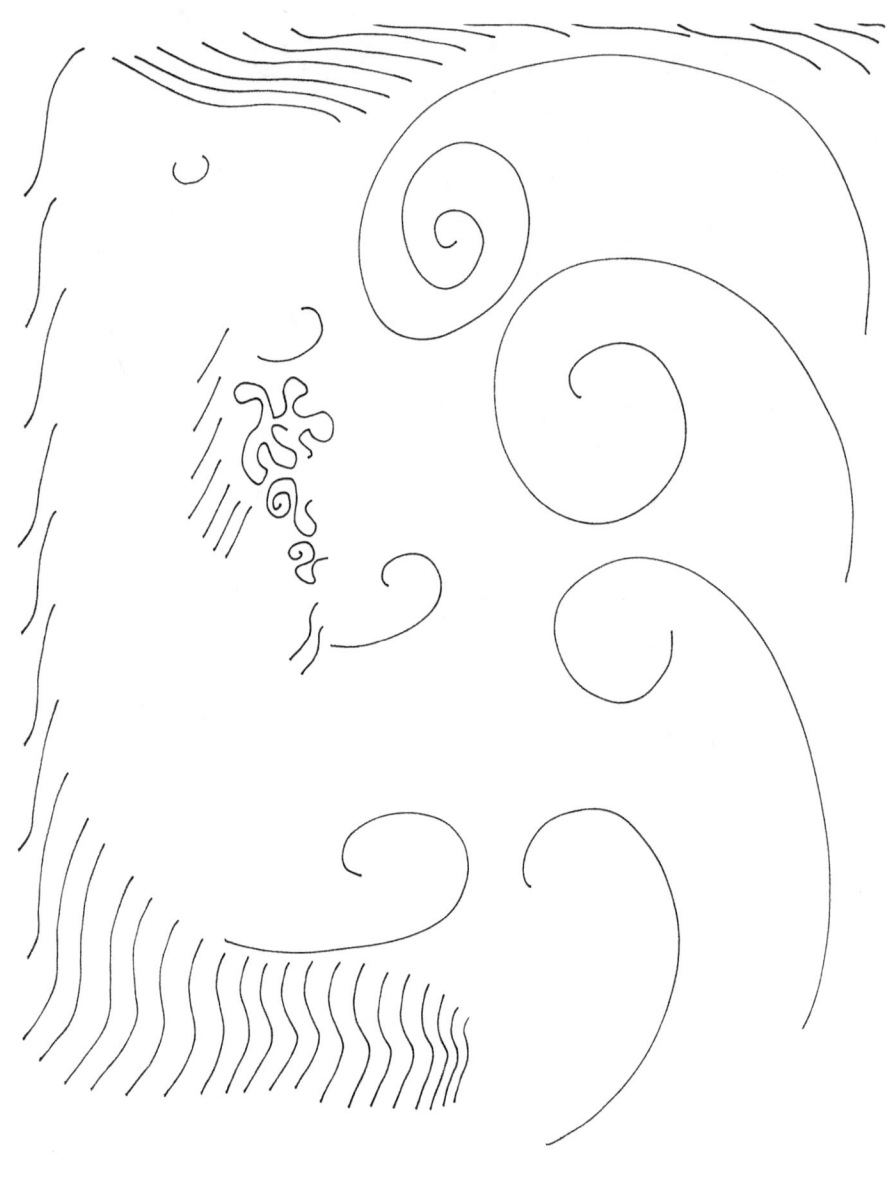

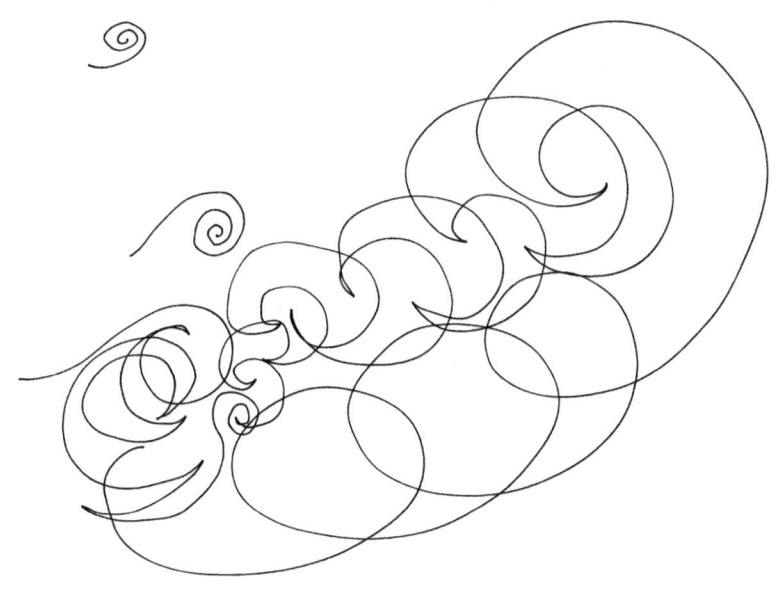

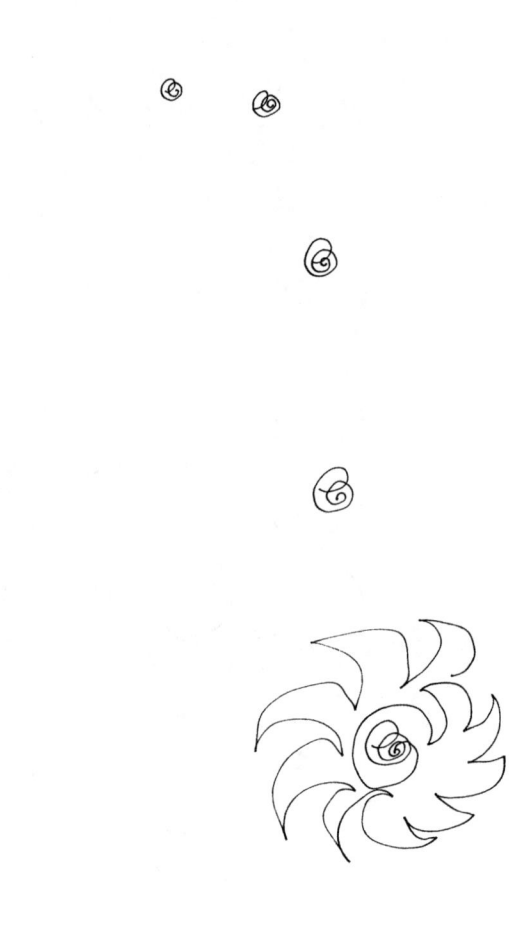

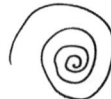
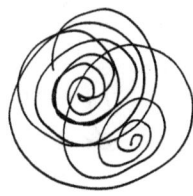

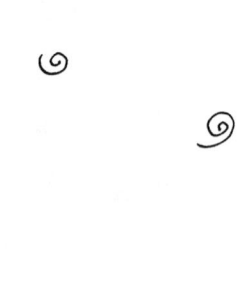
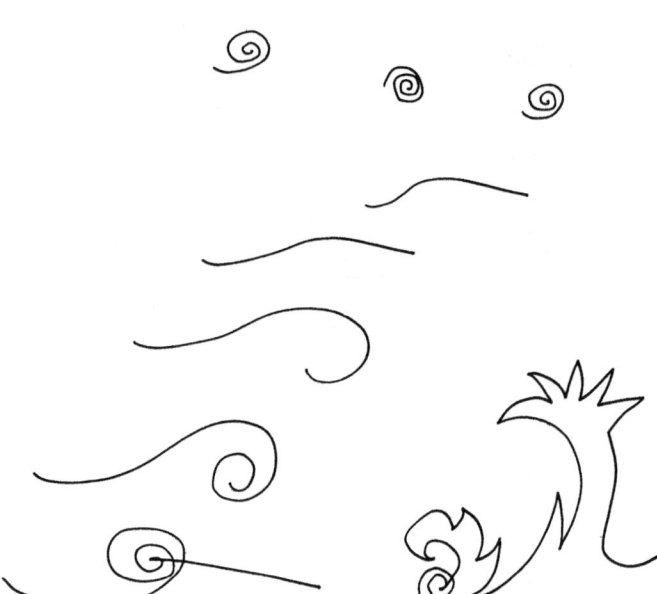

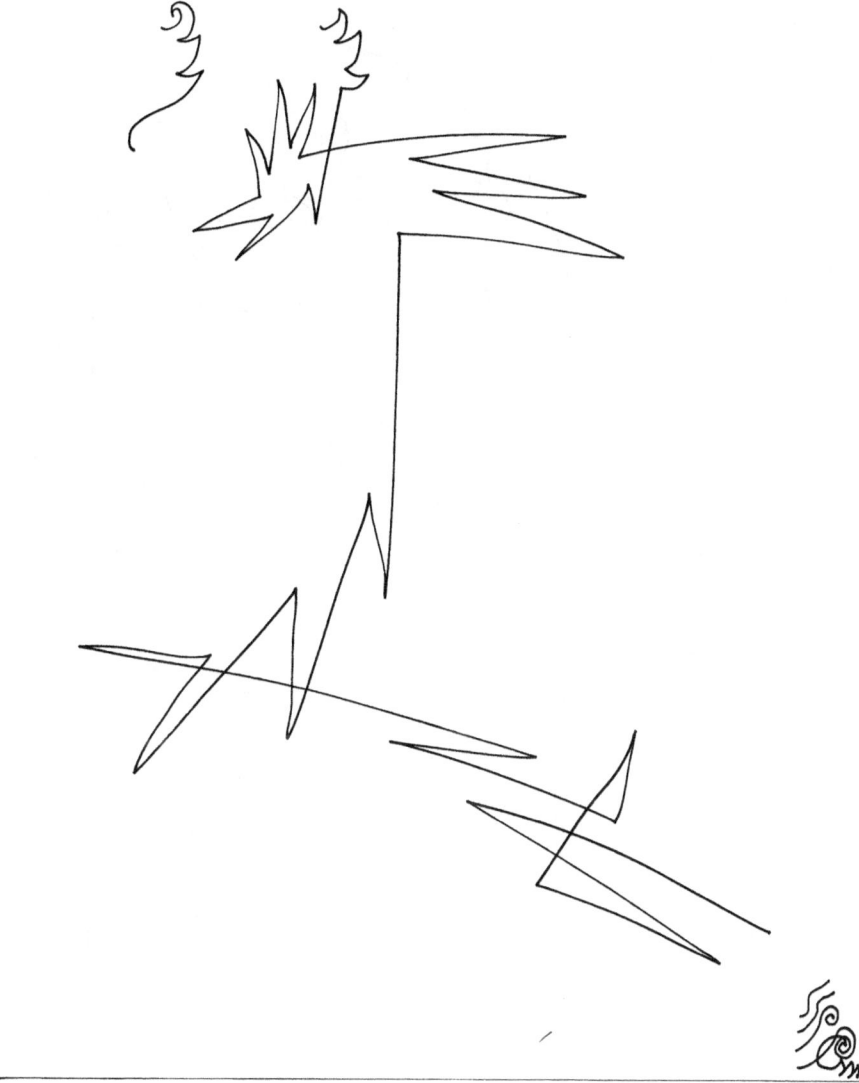

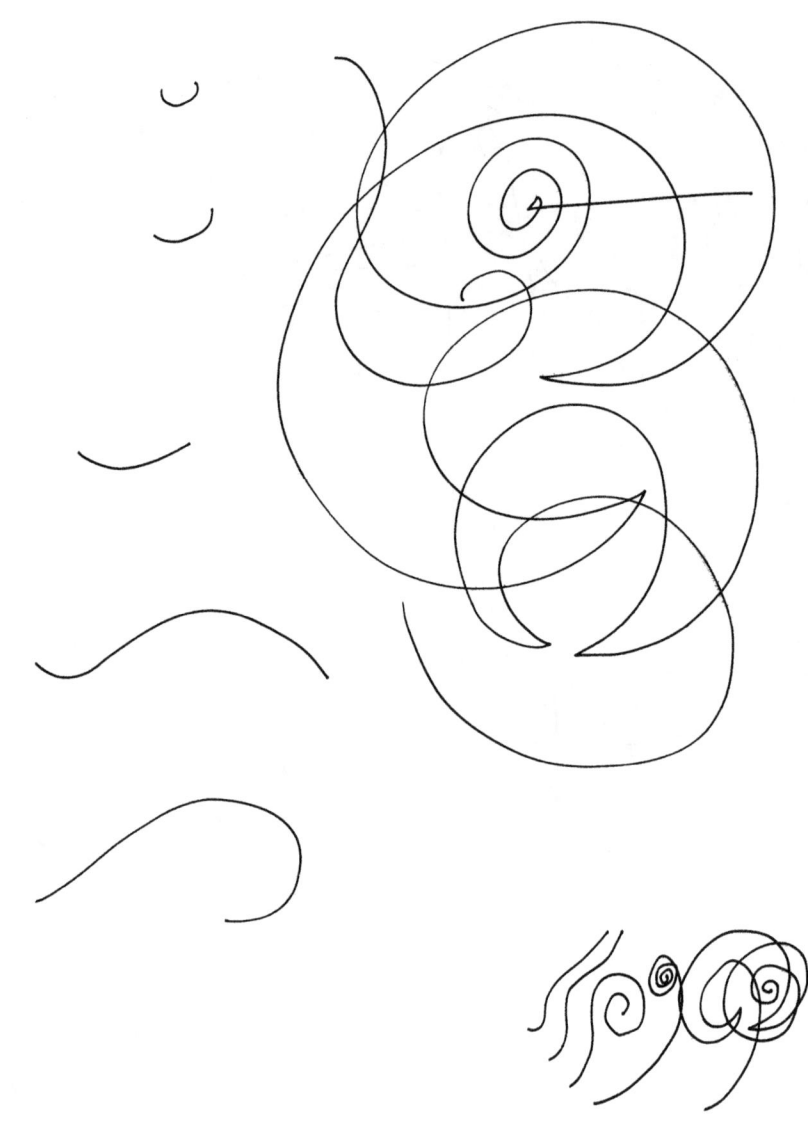

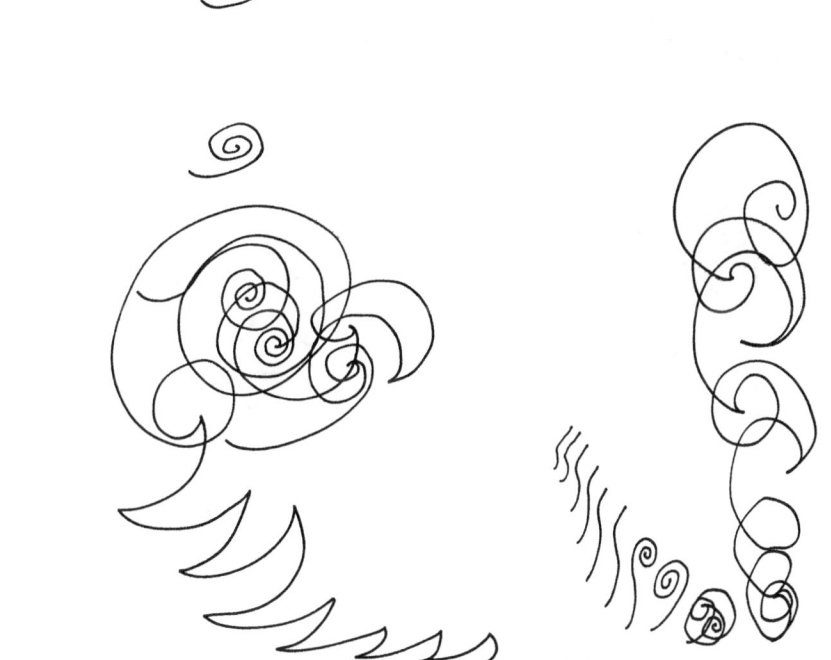

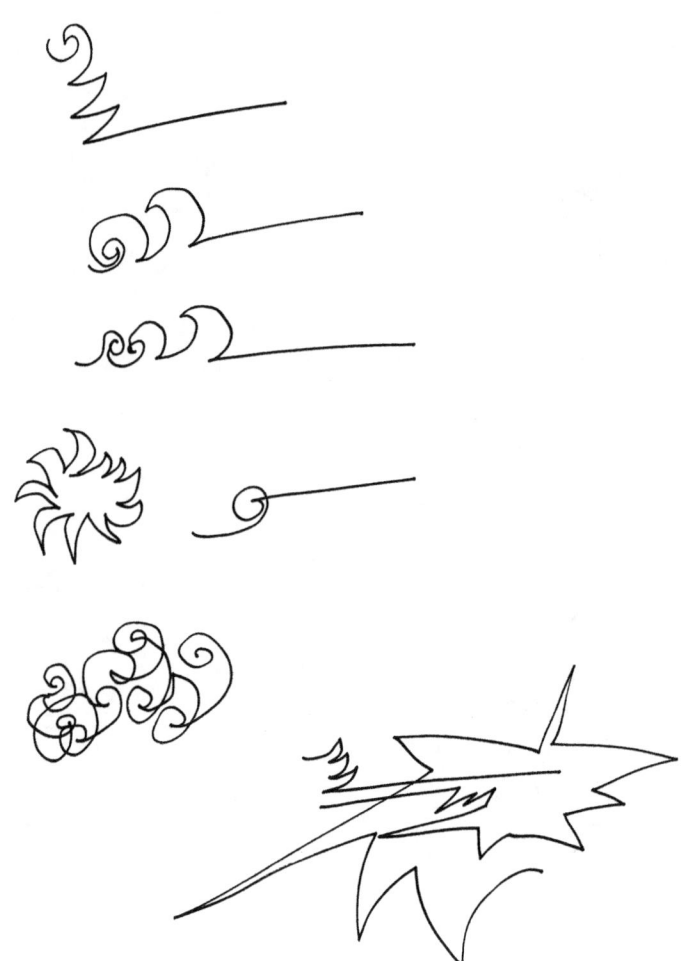

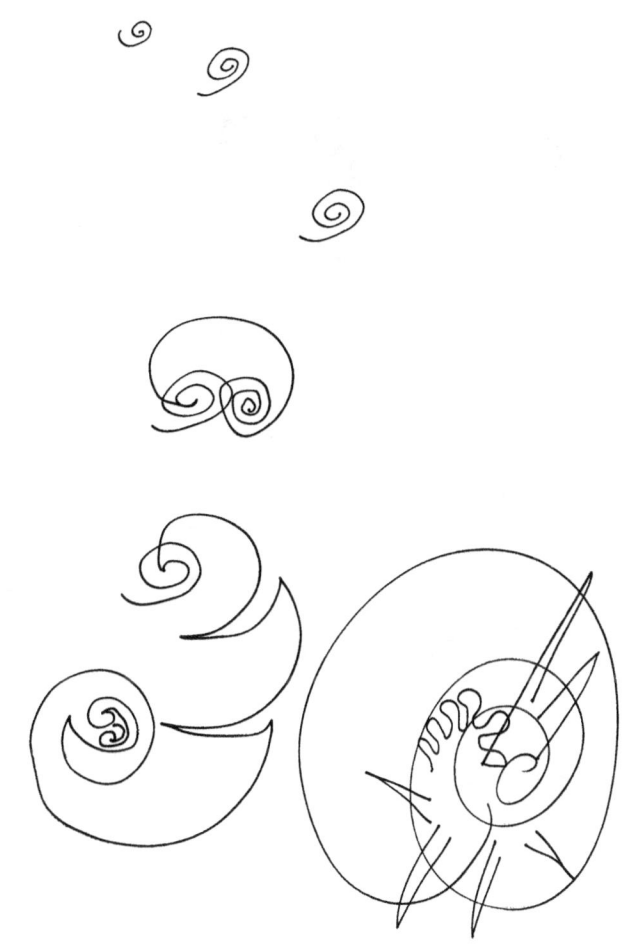

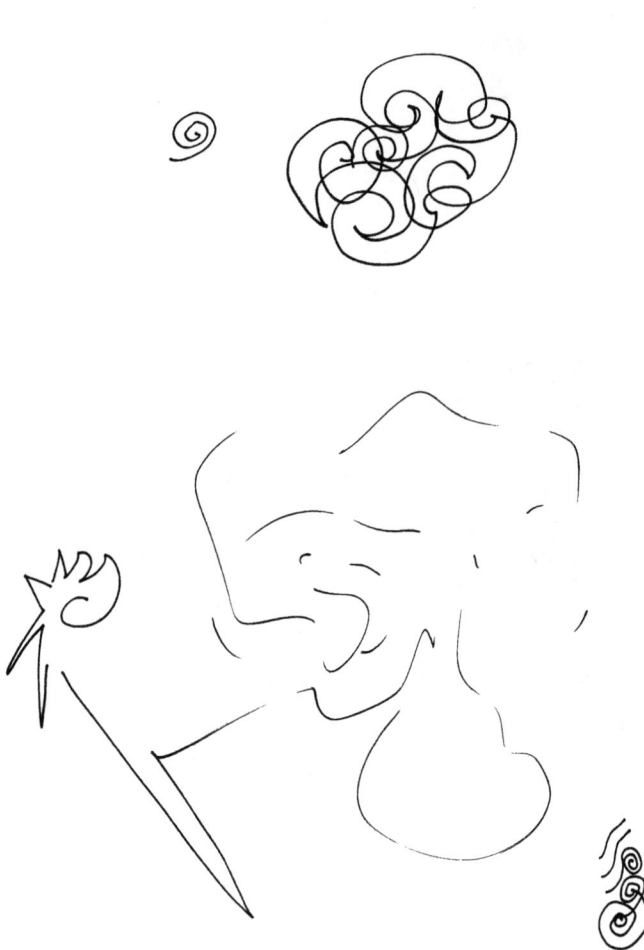

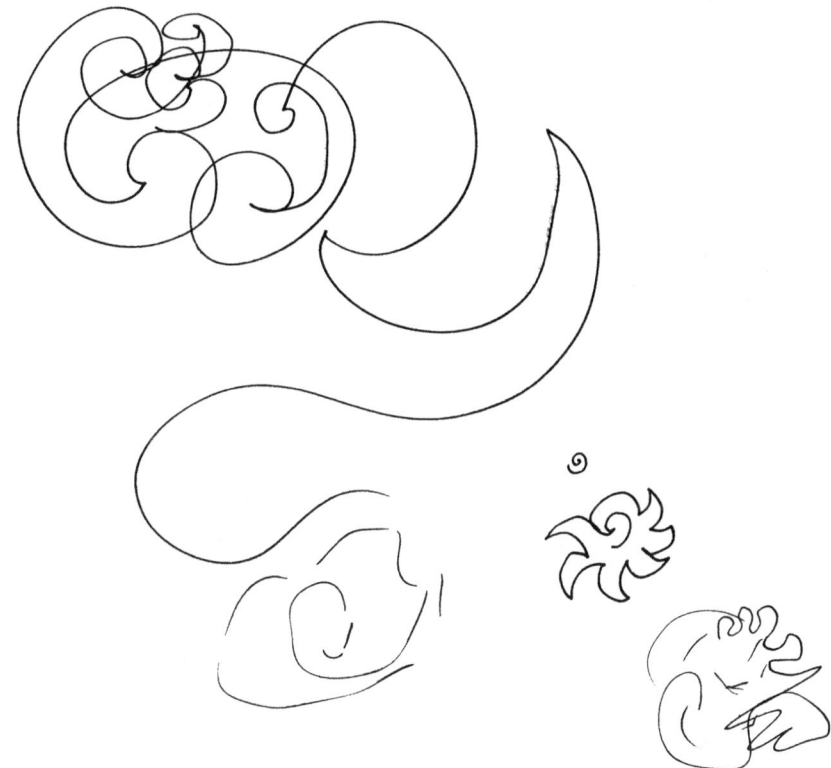

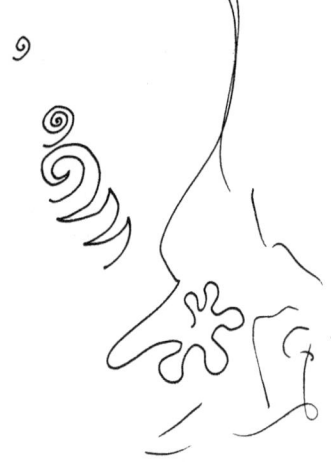

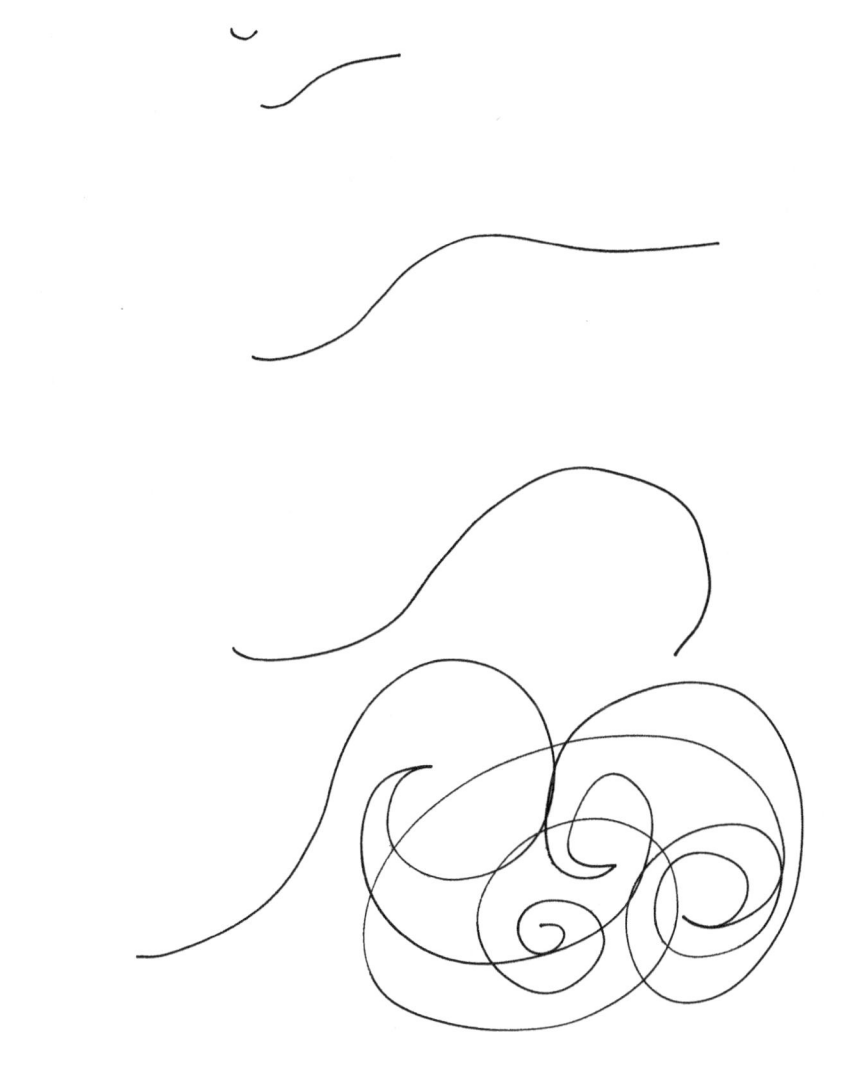

CONTINUED IN VOLUME 5